Collaborators

ROBERT J. ALPERN, M.D.

Assistant Professor of Medicine and Associate Scientist,
Cardiovascular Research Institute, University of California, San Francisco
Chapters 4 and 6

CHRISTINE A. BERRY, Ph.D.

Associate Professor of Medicine and Associate Scientist,
Cardiovascular Research Institute, University of California, San Francisco
Chapters 2 and 6

DAVID A. BUSHINSKY, M.D.

Assistant Professor of Medicine, University of Chicago Pritzker School of Medicine;
Physician, University of Chicago Hospitals and Clinics, Chicago
Chapter 7

MARTIN G. COGAN, M.D.

Associate Professor of Medicine and Associate Scientist,
Cardiovascular Research Institute, University of California, San Francisco
Chapter 5

THOMAS H. HOSTETTER, M.D.

Associate Professor of Medicine and Director, Renal Division,
University of Minnesota, Minneapolis
Chapter 3

DAVID J. LEVENSON, M.D.

Assistant Professor of Medicine, Harvard Medical School, and
Associate Physician, Brigham and Women's Hospital, Boston
Chapter 1

RENAL
PHYSIOLOGY
in Health and Disease

BARRY BRENNER, M.D.

Samuel A. Levine Professor of Medicine, Harvard Medical School;
Director, Renal Division, Brigham and Women's Hospital,
Boston, Massachusetts

FREDRIC L. COE, M.D.

Professor of Medicine and Physiology,
University of Chicago Pritzker School of Medicine;
Director, Renal Section, University of Chicago Hospitals and Clinics,
Chicago, Illinois

FLOYD C. RECTOR, Jr., M.D.

Professor of Medicine and Physiology,
Senior Scientist, Cardiovascular Research Institute,
Director, Division of Nephrology,
University of California, San Francisco, School of Medicine,
San Francisco, California

1987
W.B. SAUNDERS COMPANY
Philadelphia □ London □ Toronto □ Mexico City
Rio de Janeiro □ Sydney □ Tokyo □ Hong Kong

W. B. Saunders Company: West Washington Square
Philadelphia, PA   19105

Library of Congress Cataloging-in-Publication Data

Brenner, Barry M., 1937–

Renal physiology in health and disease.

Includes bibliographies.

1. Kidneys—Diseases.   2. Kidneys.   I. Coe, Fredric
L.   II. Rector, Floyd C., Jr.   III. Title. [DNLM: 1.
Kidney—physiology.   2. Kidney—physiopathology.
WJ 301 B838r]

RC903.9.B74 1987   616.6′1   86–3941

ISBN 0–7216–1973–8

Editor: Al Meier
Designer: Bill Donnelly
Production Manager: Bob Butler
Illustration Coordinator: Walt Verbitski
Indexer: George Vilk

Renal Physiology in Health and Disease   ISBN   0–7216–1973–8

Last digit is the print number: 9   8   7   6   5   4   3   2   1

Preface

A modest way into the hills above Cannes, not very far from Antibes, is a little town called Vallauris in which, for a time, the artist Picasso made his home. Just off the town square is the National Museum of Modern Art, housed in the Chapel of the Vallauris Castle: a monastery built in the 12th century, low to the ground, curved at the roof, and looking more like a small covered cloister than a church. Inside, its walls are hung with wooden panels on which Picasso has painted "War and Peace," his vision of mankind in its two most polar states of being. As well, one can enjoy the drawings he made as studies for the finished image; and one set of drawings, of a provincial hearse, progresses in about ten versions from its first creation to the form it takes on the panels.

The hearse starts out like a 19th century streetcar drawn by horses swinging long, showy tails. As he redrew, Picasso did what most of us would not; instead of filling in the lines, showing us surface highlights that would make us believe in the reality of the hearse, ornaments on bridles and reins, curves of horses' hooves and their rich, warm eyes, he began a process of extraction: line after line is taken away and, as if the paper could have on it only so much ink, their weights are added to the lines that remain, which become bolder and heavier. The bottom of the hearse and its three wooden extensions that join to the harnesses become massive; the delicate boxworks of the wagon condenses into a few pillars and girders; the horses elongate, legs and hooves and chests become fuller, and heads and eyes as well. The wagon becomes a chariot carrying a laconic, mindless soldier; he leans over its side holding a long, serrated sword pointing downward; three demonic horses trample books, flowers of civilization.

The problem Picasso had to solve was certainly not how to draw a hearse; the lines of the first drawing reach out for filigree to decorate themselves, and seem strong enough to guide the smudgy hands of whichever untalented school child might undertake to complete them. It was, rather, how to express his feeling about death and war through an image of a hearse become a grotesque instrument of killing; and what he did was to extract the essential structure of the wagon and the strength of the horses, and fuse them together into a metaphor, an image of something that never really has existed but can, as an image, give a physical form to his idea. The wagon and horse, elements of the real world, are transformed by the personal vision of the artist into elements of a world vision—war as death—that he embodies in image—the mural—an image that can transmit his vision to any receptive person. "When I was working on this series of drawings, I would look back over my sketchpads every day, wondering 'what am I still going to teach myself that I didn't know before?' And when it was no longer I talking, but the drawing I had done, when they had gotten away from me and were defying me, then I knew I'd reached my goal. . ."*

All paintings are metaphors in a sense, as their few lines must stand for the overpowering detail of reality; even a photograph is metaphor, a wedge cut out of life and flattened onto a page. In the same way, teaching and explanations of natural things are metaphors, too: stories we tell each other about incomprehensible masses of detail. What is remarkable about the wagon is that the drawings, the acts of conversion, are not hidden and secret, the transmogrification is carried to an extreme, and the final result is washed over with such beauty as to endear it to mankind and ensure it will always be loved and protected. But the process is the same in acts of lesser consequence, whenever image or words must stand against the intolerable density of real life.

Our two books, this one and its mate, stand somewhere closer to the end of the drawings than the beginning. At the beginning, just at the point that elements of the real world are transferred to paper, is the research report: what living people see becomes numbers and drawings and photographs; some few lines of the real world are defined well enough that everyone can agree on their shapes. Actual perception is reduced to symbols on a page, and in the transformation much of the truth is irretrievably lost. At the end, the perceived elements of the real world become elements of a scientific world vision, that exists in the minds of some scientists and sometimes is made explicit in texts, and concerns such matters as how cells and organs work, why people are ill, how they may be cured, and the manners and the times of their deaths. In between is the chain of explanations, the paring away of details to disclose the elements of structure they hide and complicate, all of it guided by visions of what is, of how things really are, of the nature of illness and the workings of our craft. Usually the personal vision of a single artist is replaced by the collective and shared vision of many scientists, who each contribute only a few fragments. Occasionally, one person creates the vision, compelling and perfect, and communicates it to the world; we find ourselves in the company of genius, like Picasso, but in a person of science.

In order to place our two volumes properly along the chain of explanations we spokesmen for a shared and collective vision need to contrive a kind of ruler, a sequence of benchmarks from observation to synthetic vision. Perhaps the first step after the research report is the review, the long analytical discursion all of us have committed from time to time: every paper noted down, conflicts played out number on number, method on method, judged by simple matters of shopwork—who is most accurate in drawing their lines, most consistent, and therefore most believable? After the review must surely come the encyclopedias, the multiauthored and unconquerable behemoths that roll over lesser works, push them aside, and station themselves at

---

*Cabanne, P.: Pablo Picasso—His Life and Times. Morrow, New York, 1971, p 427.

every crossroad that people must pass on the way to learning. Just before the end must be those works that are truly synthetic, that create the vision without its obscuring elements for anyone to read; probably there are few such writings, and most by single authors who have struggled enough that they have achieved a coherent image of the world. Between the behemoths and the solitary vision, we hope closer to the latter, are our two volumes, which we three have written in our middle years, aided in selected chapters by a few close and highly regarded younger colleagues.

Why write them at all? Partly for ". . . ambition or bread/ Or the strut and trade of charms/ On the ivory stages";* perhaps as useful advice for tourists in the puzzling land of the kidney; certainly because writing is a pleasure beyond words. Most of all, because we have looked on the realities of renal disease and physiology long enough to draw the details lifelike, fully, and enjoy the conversion of detail into vision. In *Renal Physiology in Health and Disease,* we have written about the main things the kidneys do: filter, reabsorb, and secrete sodium, potassium, hydrogen, and water; make hormones; regulate the volume, pressure, and composition of the blood. We have taken away the details that are not structural, so the ways things work are easier to understand. In our companion volume on *Clinical Nephrology* we write about how the kidneys are injured, how their cells may die, how we come to realize that such things are happening, and how we may contrive a treatment for the kidneys or for the patient who has lost them. The clinical volume is not enough for a consultant, but is right for students, housestaff, and doctors who want to understand nephrology even though it is not their special interest.

Perhaps in honor of the Chapel of Vallauris we have not signed the chapters; like medieval scholars we leave authorship as a simple puzzle for our friends. We do acknowledge the help that our colleagues have given us, substantial help indeed in the labor of collecting and sifting the details from which we have selected the texts. In homage to the Chapel, and its grand possessions, we have done our best to present our thoughts in workmanlike phrases; for beauty is beyond us who work in our humble craft, and even unseemly for cataloging the miseries of illness which are our chief concern. But even so there is a grandeur in all of nature, which graces medicine and its pursuits just as it does the world from which all art must ultimately arise; and as best we can we have written by its light.

---

*Thomas, D.: Collected Poems. Laughlin, New York, 1953, p 142.

Contents

Structure and Function of the Renal Circulations

Maintenance of a stable internal milieu is essential for survival of all creatures. For mammals, the necessary features of such an internal environment include appropriate oxygen and carbon dioxide tensions, body temperature, energy stores, and body fluid volume and composition. In this context the primary role of the kidney is to ensure the near-constancy of the extracellular fluid. It accomplishes these tasks by regulating the volume and composition of fluid excreted as urine, so as to compensate for varying intake of food and water, for non-renal losses of fluid and electrolytes (in sweat, stool, etc.), and for the continual but variable production of metabolic waste products. Thus, the kidney is able to modulate the excretion of water, sodium, potassium, calcium, magnesium, chloride, phosphate, hydrogen, and bicarbonate ions, among others, while limiting urinary losses of essential plasma proteins, glucose, and other organic substances and, at the same time, promoting the elimination of waste products such as urea and creatinine. This chapter considers the role of the various elements of the renal circulation in facilitating these physiologic functions. As will become apparent, blood flow to the kidneys serves these ends in three ways: (1) by supplying the nutrients, oxygen, and metabolic substrates necessary for renal cell function; (2) by delivering, in the plasma water, the unneeded solutes destined for excretion into urine; and (3) by participating in, and regulating, the processes of glomerular filtration, tubule fluid and ion reabsorption and secretion, and urine concentration and dilution, the central events in urine formation.

ANATOMY OF THE RENAL VASCULATURE

The renal arteries diverge from the upper abdominal aorta just below the origins of the celiac axis and superior mesenteric artery. Within the renal hilum, and just before entering the parenchyma, the main *renal artery* divides into *anterior* and *posterior branches* (Fig. 1–1). The anterior branch divides further into approximately four *segmental* arteries which together supply some two thirds of the kidney tissue, including both poles. Segmental divisions of the posterior branch provide perfusion to the posterior surface of the kidney. Within the medulla the segmental arteries divide into *interlobar* arteries, which ascend toward the cortex within the renal columns of Bertin. At the corticomedullary junction branches of the interlobar vessels course parallel to the renal surface as *arcuate arteries*, then divide and ascend perpendicularly toward the renal capsule as *interlobular arteries* (Fig. 1–2). *Afferent arterioles* branch directly from these vessels, carrying blood to *glomerular capillaries* distributed throughout the cortex. This capillary network represents the first of several microcirculations to be encountered in the process of blood transit through the kidney. Thus, cells and plasma exit the glomerular microcirculation in *efferent arterioles* (rather than venules). The subsequent intrarenal circulatory route depends upon the cortical location of the glomeruli from which the

Efferent arterioles lead from glomerular capillaries to three separate postglomerular capillary beds: cortical, outer medullary, and inner medullary (vasa recta).

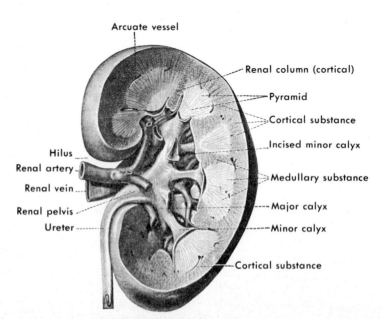

Arcuate vessel

Renal column (cortical)
Pyramid
Cortical substance
Incised minor calyx
Hilus
Renal artery
Renal vein
Medullary substance
Renal pelvis
Major calyx
Ureter
Minor calyx

Cortical substance

Figure 1–1. Anatomy of the human kidney, posterior view. (From Bloom, W., and Fawcett, D. W.: A Textbook of Histology, 10th Edition. W. B. Saunders Co., Philadelphia, 1975, with permission.)

efferent arterioles exit: mid and outer cortical glomeruli give rise to the postglomerular, cortical peritubular capillary microcirculation, whereas efferent arterioles from deeper glomeruli descend into the medulla. There they provide both the outer medullary peritubular capillary microcirculation and the *vasa recta*, which accompany thin limbs of Henle's loops into the inner medulla. The nature and physiologic importance of these separate intrarenal capillary beds is discussed in further detail in subsequent sections of this chapter.

The true venous circulation of the kidney begins as blood exits the capillaries of the peritubular networks and the vasa recta. Venules from regions throughout the cortex merge into *interlobular veins* and descend toward the corticomedullary junction, where they are joined by veins draining the medullary microcirculations. The subsequent pattern of *arcuate, interlobar,* and *segmental veins* is similar to that found in the arterial circulation, except for the presence of multiple anastomoses between veins at all levels of the venous circulation.

. It is apparent from this description that renal vascular anatomy is highly organized, particularly when contrasted to many other organs where capillary beds are distributed randomly throughout the tissue and provide direct and short distance connections between their perfusing and draining vessels. However, the seemingly anomalous features of the renal microcirculations take on a highly rational basis when one views them in terms of the intimate anatomic relationships that exist between microvascular and nephron structures within the kidney. Indeed, the specialized structural properties of the various renal microcirculations facilitate function at each step in the process of urine formation. Thus, the glomerular microcirculation has properties uniquely suited to ultrafiltration, the cortical peritubular capillary network to the reabsorption and secretion of filtered fluid and solutes, and the medullary circulations to urine concentration and dilution. Furthermore, the anatomic proximity of tubule and capillary permits the Starling forces (hydraulic and oncotic pressures) which exist across the walls of the capillaries to exert an important effect on tubule fluid transport processes. In this manner capillary hemodynamics provide an extremely effective mechanism by which the renal vasculature ultimately regulates the volume and composition of the final urine.

Renal Capillaries and Their Functions

Glomerular:
Ultrafiltration

Cortical:
Reabsorption and secretion

Medullary:
Reabsorption and secretion, urine concentration and dilution

RENAL HEMODYNAMICS AND REGULATION OF RENAL VASCULAR TONE

The two kidneys of a typical 70-kg person together weigh approximately 300 gm, or about 0.4 percent of total body weight. They receive blood flow at the rate of 1.2 liters/min or about one fifth of resting cardiac output. This rate of tissue perfusion, 4 ml/min/gm tissue, is much higher than in other well-perfused organs such as heart, liver, and brain (Table 1–1). Most of this flow supplies the metabolically active renal cortex, whereas 10 percent of renal blood flow (RBF) is directed toward the outer medulla and only 1 to 2 percent into the papillary tissue. Although the deeper areas are relatively ischemic, the flow per gram of tissue in these regions is in fact quite comparable to that of other well-perfused organs. Further evidence that tissue per-

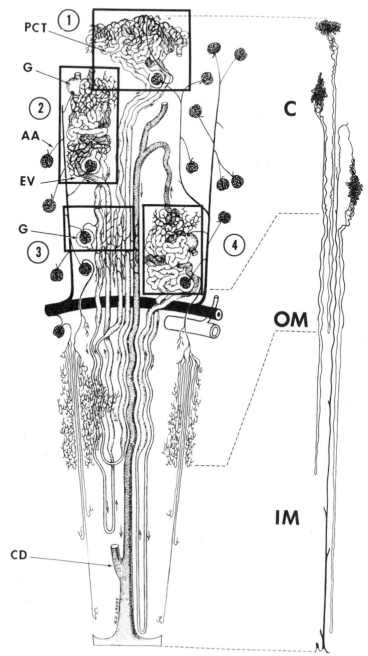

Figure 1–2. *See legend on opposite page.*

Table 1–1. BLOOD FLOW RATES AND OXYGEN CONSUMPTION
RATES OF SEVERAL ORGANS IN HUMANS

Organ	Mass (gm)	Blood Flow Rate (ml/100 gm/min)	Arteriovenous Oxygen Concentration Difference (μ moles/100 ml)	Oxygen Consumption Rate (μ moles/100 gm/min)
Kidney	300	420	63	267
Brain	1,400	54	276	147
Skin	3,600	13	111	15
Skeletal muscle	31,000	3	267	7
Heart	300	84	508	431

fusion is relatively luxurious in the kidney is derived from the rate of oxygen uptake, measured as the arteriovenous oxygen concentration difference. As shown in Table 1–1, only a small percentage of the supplied oxygen is extracted, in contrast to heart, brain, and skeletal muscle. But because blood flow rate is so high, renal oxygen consumption per gram of tissue is exceeded only by heart muscle.

Values for RBF in women are somewhat lower than for men when corrected for body surface area (980 vs. 1200 ml/min/1.73 m²) but are equal when normalized for kidney weight. Maximum values for RBF are reached at age 20 to 30 and decline gradually to about 60 percent of maximum in octogenarians. A variety of factors are capable of increasing RBF chronically. In normal pregnancy RBF may rise by about 40 percent, in part because of the influence of gestational hormones. When one kidney is removed, because of disease or trauma, blood flow to the remaining kidney usually doubles over the course of weeks. Such a functional reserve capacity permits maintenance of essential renal functions despite loss of half of renal mass. Dietary protein intake also stimulates RBF, both acutely and under more chronic circumstances.

Figure 1–2. Diagram showing the vascular and tubule organization of the kidney in the dog (C, cortex; OM, outer medulla; IM, inner medulla). At the right, drawn to scale, are nephrons arising from glomeruli in outer, middle, and inner cortex. At left, tubule and vascular relations are illustrated schematically. An arcuate artery lying at the corticomedullary junction gives rise to interlobular arteries which ascend toward the cortical surface, branching info afferent arterioles (AA) that supply individual glomeruli (G). The efferent vessels (EV) from these glomeruli divide to form the peritubular capillaries. At the kidney surface (rectangle 1), proximal convoluted tubules (PCT) are associated with a dense capillary network arising from division of superficial efferent arterioles. In the middle and inner cortex (rectangles 2 and 4), convoluted tubule segments are located close to interlobular arteries and are perfused by a complex peritubular capillary network usually derived from the efferent vessels of many glomeruli. Midway between interlobular vessels, loops of Henle are grouped together with collecting ducts (CD) as medullary rays. The peritubular capillary network of this region (rectangle 3), derived from midcortical efferent arterioles, provides perfusion to the tubule structures of the medullary ray. In the inner or juxtamedullary cortex (rectangle 4), glomeruli have efferent arterioles that descend and divide to form outer medullary vascular bundles. A dense outer medullary capillary network arises from these bundles. Only thin limbs of Henle extend with collecting ducts to the papillary tip. These are accompanied by vasa recta extending from the cores of the vascular bundles. For simplicity, venous vessels have not been shown. (From Brenner, B. M., and Rector, F. C., Jr., eds.: The Kidney, 3rd Edition. W. B. Saunders Co., Philadelphia, 1986, with permission.)

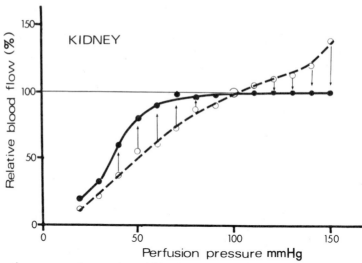

Figure 1–3. Autoregulation of renal blood flow in the dog kidney. The transient blood flow rate following alterations in renal perfusion pressure is shown as a dashed line, and the flow rate obtained under steady-state conditions is depicted as a solid line. At perfusion pressures above 60 to 70 mm Hg, steady-state renal blood flow is relatively constant. (From Brenner, B. M., and Rector, F. C., Jr., eds.: The Kidney, 3rd Edition. W. B. Saunders Co., Philadelphia, 1986, with permission.)

Autoregulation is a term used to describe the relative constancy of GFR and RBF that occurs in response to variations in perfusion pressure.

Autoregulation. Renal vascular tone is dynamic and responds rapidly to a variety of stimuli, including changes in the pressure of the perfusing blood. If renal artery perfusion pressure declines, renal vessels dilate to minimize the local impact of the reduction in RBF (Fig. 1–3). This effect is most evident above 50 to 60 mm Hg; below this range further vasodilation does not occur, and RBF declines in proportion to the reduction in perfusion pressure. *Autoregulation* of RBF is related to the influence of a number of vasoactive hormones as well as to the ability of arterioles in general to respond to *tangential wall tension*. The latter mechanism, often referred to as a *myogenic reflex*, reduces vessel wall tone within seconds as transmural pressure declines, or increases wall tone just as rapidly when renal perfusion pressure rises abruptly. This reflex appears to be an intrinsic property of the vessel wall: it persists after renal denervation or interruption of renal hormone systems but is abolished by agents which paralyze smooth muscle contraction. Autoregulation of glomerular filtration rate (GFR) is also seen with changes in renal perfusion pressure, mediated by vascular resistance mechanisms which are described below.

Hormonal and Neural Control. Renal vascular tone is affected by neural impulses and by circulating and intrarenal vasoactive compounds. The primary sites at which these factors influence intrarenal vascular resistance are the *afferent* and *efferent arterioles*. In addition, medium-sized arteries, glomerular mesangial cells, and the smooth muscle cells in the walls of postglomerular medullary vessels contain contractile elements which may also be responsive to vasocontrictor and vasodilator hormones. Neural and hormonal influences are the fundamental regulators of the renal circulations and indirectly modify a host of intrarenal transport functions. The general features of these hormonal and neural systems are described here, and their specific effects on glomerular and peritubular microcirculations are discussed in corresponding sections of this chapter.

Renin-Angiotensin-Aldosterone System. The renin-angiotensin-aldosterone system (RAAS) is an important regulator of renal and systemic hemodynamics, and participates in the maintenance of salt and water balance (Fig. 1–4). The kidney releases into the circulation a proteolytic enzyme, *renin*. The action of renin upon its hepatically synthesized tetradecapeptide substrate, *angiotensinogen*, produces a relatively inactive decapeptide, *angiotensin I* (AI). Removal from AI of two terminal amino acids occurs primarily within the pulmonary circulation by the action of *angiotensin I converting enzyme* and forms the potently vasoactive octapeptide, *angiotensin II* (AII).

AII has two major physiologic effects: (1) on a molar basis it is one of the most potent vasoconstrictor substances known, and (2) it is a specific stimulator of release of the sodium-retaining hormone *aldosterone* by the adrenal cortex. Together these two effects serve to raise blood pressure and increase intravascular volume, essential protective mechanisms activated to defend circulatory homeostasis in states of hypotension or perceived volume loss. The specific intrarenal effects of AII on GFR, fluid reabsorption, and sodium balance are considered below and in Chapter 3.

Renin is stored primarily within the granules of specialized myoepithelial cells (*juxtaglomerular cells*) located in the walls of renal afferent arterioles (Fig. 1–5). The rate of its release into the renal

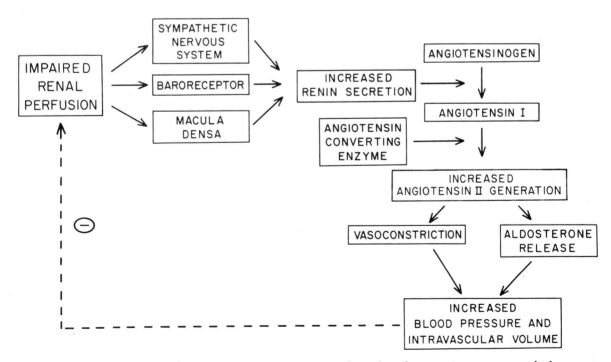

Figure 1–4. The renin-angiotensin-aldosterone system. Impaired renal perfusion activates sensors which promote renin release, stimulating the production of angiotensin II and aldosterone. The resulting vasoconstriction and sodium retention increase blood pressure and intravascular volume, returning renal perfusion toward normal.

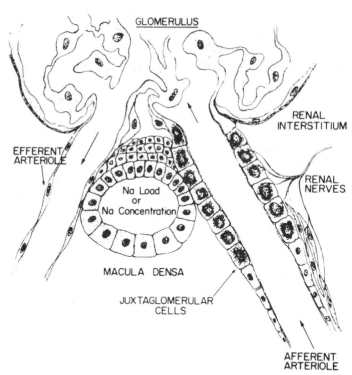

Figure 1–5. Anatomic relationships of intrarenal effectors of renin release. Juxtaglomerular cells of the afferent arteriole release renin in response to reduced perfusion pressure, renal sympathetic nerve stimulation, or altered delivery of sodium to the macula densa portion of the distal tubule. The close anatomic proximity of efferent arteriole and glomerulus is evident. (From Davis, J. O.: What signals the kidney to release renin? Circ. Res. 28:301–306, 1971, with permission.)

Renin release is augmented by
- *Reduced perfusion pressure*
- *β-adrenergic stimulation*
- *Reduced NaCl concentration in macula densa*
- *Chronic hypokalemia*

Renin release is inhibited by
- *Increased perfusion pressure*
- *AII acting directly*
- *Atrial peptides*

venous plasma is a major determinant of ambient AII levels, and this release is dependent upon at least three intrarenal sensing mechanisms. Reduction in renal perfusion pressure or alterations in arterial wall tension stimulates renin release, the so-called *renal baroreceptor* mechanism (Fig. 1–4). Acute hypotension and chronic renal artery stenosis are clinical examples of such stimuli. The sympathetic nervous system as well as circulating catecholamines also provoke renin release through an independent process dependent upon β-*adrenergic receptors*. This pathway accounts, in part, for the renin secretory response to acute hypotension, upright posture, chronic salt depletion, and exercise. However, β-adrenergic receptor blockade with propranolol only partially inhibits renin release under these conditions, indicating that other mechanisms are capable of augmenting renin secretion. The composition of fluid delivered to the distal tubule also influences the rate of renin release. Specialized cells of the thick ascending limb of Henle's loop (the *macula densa*) lie in juxtaposition to the glomerulus and its afferent and efferent arterioles. These cells detect changes in the composition of the fluid delivered to the macula densa, such that a fall in NaCl concentration promotes renin release.

The net consequences of augmented renin release, namely increased intravascular volume, elevated blood pressure, and improved renal perfusion, constitute a negative feedback mechanism for suppressing further renin release (Fig. 1–4). Evidence for direct inhibition of renin release by AII also exists (the so-called *short feedback loop*). This is apparently a direct effect of AII on juxtaglomerular cells, independent of changes in renal hemodynamics. In addition, acute hypernatremia inhibits, and chronic hypokalemia stimulates, renin release.

Renal Nerves and Circulating Catecholamines. The kidney is richly innervated with fibers from the celiac plexus and other sources within the abdomen and thorax. These provide innervation to major intrarenal arteries, afferent arterioles, and, to a lesser extent, glomerular mesangium, efferent arterioles, and tubule structures. In addition to the indirect effect of β-*adrenergic stimulation* to alter renal vascular tone through activation of the renin-angiotensin system, renal sympathetic nerves and circulating catecholamines exert other important regulatory influences on the renal circulation. Direct α-*adrenergic stimulation* of the kidney produces marked vasoconstriction and a fall in RBF. However, under basal conditions renal neural stimulation is low, and denervation or blockade of α receptors under this circumstance has little influence on renal function. In contrast, hemorrhage, anesthesia, heart failure, pain, and conditions which provoke the "fright or flight" response can induce neurally mediated vasoconstriction. Dopamine may be another endogenous renal neurotransmitter, acting upon specific receptors to induce renal vasodilation.

Prostaglandins. Renal prostaglandins and thromboxane are potent vasoactive metabolites of arachidonic acid. They are produced locally

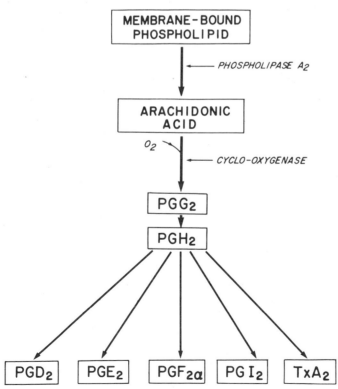

Figure 1–6. Pathways for synthesis of prostaglandins and thromboxane A_2 (TxA_2). Release of arachidonic acid by phospholipase A_2 is the rate-limiting step. (Modified from Levenson, D. J., et al.: Arachidonic acid metabolism, prostaglandins and the kidney. Am. J. Med. 72:354–374, 1982, with permission.)

through a mechanism which is stimulated by renal vasoconstrictors (AII, norepinephrine, vasopressin, α-adrenergic neural stimulation) and inhibited by cyclo-oxygenase inhibitors such as aspirin, indomethacin, and other nonsteroidal anti-inflammatory agents (NSAIDs) (Fig. 1–6). The primary vasoactive intrarenal endproducts of arachidonate metabolism are the vasodilators PGE_2 and PGI_2 (prostacyclin); thromboxane A_2 (TxA_2), a potent vasoconstrictor, is produced to a lesser extent, although certain conditions such as ureteral obstruction can

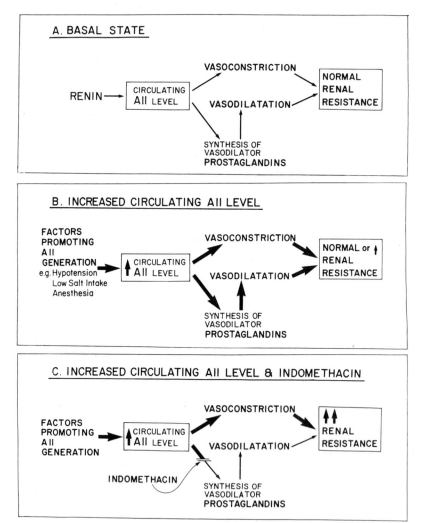

Figure 1–7. Interactions of angiotensin II (AII) and prostaglandins in the regulation of renal vascular resistance. Circulating AII directly promotes renal vasoconstriction, and also stimulates production of vasodilator prostaglandins, which oppose the constrictor effects of AII. Under basal conditions (panel A) both AII and prostaglandin levels are low, exerting minimal effects on renal vascular tone. When renin release is stimulated (panel B), elevated ambient AII levels exert two counterbalancing effects on renal resistance: a direct vasoconstrictor action on renal vessels and a stimulation of vasodilator prostaglandin synthesis. AII-induced changes in renal vascular resistance are thus minimized. During states of AII excess and concomitant blockade of prostaglandin synthesis (panel C), an exaggerated increase in renal vascular resistance results from the unopposed vasoconstrictor action of AII. (From Levenson, D. J., et al.: Arachidonic acid metabolism, prostaglandins and the kidney. Am. J. Med. 72:354–374, 1982, with permission.)

markedly augment its synthesis. Other metabolites (PGD_2 and $PGF_{2\alpha}$) are relatively inactive.

Under basal conditions the products of arachidonate metabolism are present at low levels and exert little influence on the renal circulation (Fig. 1–7, upper panel). However, when renal vasoconstrictor forces are activated (as in hypovolemia, chronic sodium depletion, congestive heart failure, or cirrhosis), vasodilator prostaglandin synthesis is augmented, counterbalancing these vasoconstrictor forces and minimizing the decline in RBF which might otherwise ensue (Fig. 1–7, middle panel). When aspirin or related drugs are administered under such conditions, marked reductions in RBF are observed, demonstrating loss of the protective effect of prostaglandins on renal hemodynamics (Fig. 1–7, lower panel). Because GFR and tubule fluid reabsorption depend on the appropriate balance of intrarenal vascular resistances, alterations in RBF produced by inhibition of prostaglandin synthesis result in disruption of these processes as well (see below).

Other Vasoactive Renal Hormones. The *kinins* are potent renal vasodilator substances released from inert precursor kininogens by the action of the proteolytic enzyme *kallikrein* (Fig. 1–8). Circulating kallikrein, when activated by Hageman factor (factor XIII) and other stimuli, produces the circulating kinin, *bradykinin*, whereas tissue ("glandular") kallikrein, which is activated by other factors, yields *kallidin*. Although potent renal vascular effects can be produced by intrarenal infusion of kinins, controversy surrounds the possible physiologic role of these hormones in maintaining vessel tone under normal and pathophysiologic conditions. Interactions of kinins with the RAAS and prostaglandins have been demonstrated experimentally, but their

Renal vasoconstrictors:
- *AII*
- *α-adrenergic stimulation*
- *TxA₂*
- *Norepinephrine*
- *Vasopressin*

Renal vasodilators:
- *PGE₂*
- *PGI₂*
- *Kinins*
- *Atrial peptides*

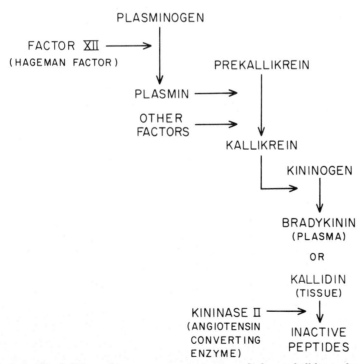

Figure 1–8. The kallikrein-kinin system. Activation of plasma kallikrein by plasmin occurs in plasma, leading to production of bradykinin. In the kidney, stimulation of glandular kallikrein by other factors yields kallidin.

significance remains uncertain. A number of other hormones, including *histamine, serotonin, acetylcholine,* and *parathyroid hormone,* have renal vasoactive properties, but once again their contributions, if any, to the control of RBF in health and disease are unknown. Finally, peptides synthesized, stored and released from atrial myocytes have been shown to exert vasorelaxant as well as natriuretic and diuretic properties. The predominant circulating peptide contains 28 amino acids and is released in response to atrial stretch, a stimulus induced by central blood volume expansion.

Pharmacologic Renal Vasodilation. *Captopril* effectively interrupts the RAAS by blocking angiotensin I converting enzyme activity. The same enzyme, also called kininase II, degrades kinins, so that its inhibition by captopril is a second mechanism of action. *Saralasin* is a specific AII receptor antagonist.

THE GLOMERULAR MICROCIRCULATION

Mechanisms of Ultrafiltration. The first step in urine formation occurs in the *glomerulus,* a structure consisting of a dense cluster of capillaries situated in the proximal end of the renal tubule (Bowman's capsule) (Fig. 1–9). The glomerular capillary wall consists of three discrete regions: the fenestrated capillary endothelium, an acellular basement membrane area, and an overlying layer of specialized epithelial cells, or podocytes, which display a complex pattern of interdigitating foot processes or pedicels (Fig. 1–10). Although the GFR per glomerulus [single nephron GFR (SNGFR)] is only about 60 nl/min in

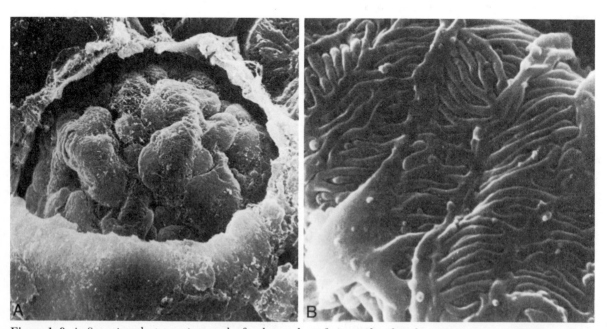

Figure 1–9. A. Scanning electron micrograph of a glomerular tuft situated within the urinary space, with the overlying Bowman's capsule broken away. B. Higher magnification, demonstrating epithelial cells with interdigitating foot processes covering the outer surface of a glomerular capillary loop. (From Brenner, B. M., and Beeuwkes, R., III: The renal circulations. Hosp. Prac. 13:35–46, 1978, with permission.)

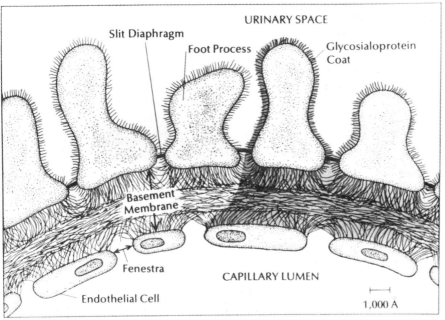

Figure 1–10. Glomerular capillary wall in cross-section. The luminal surface is covered by fenestrated endothelial cells. The basement membrane has a middle lamina densa, surrounded by lamina rara interna and externa. Overlying this are the foot processes of epithelial cells, separated by small slit diaphragms. Regions with anionic glycosialoproteins are shown in grey tone. (Illustration by Nancy Lou Gahan Markris; from Brenner, B. M., and Beeuwkes, R., III: The renal circulations. Hosp. Prac. 13:35–46, 1978, with permission.)

humans, it is much higher per unit surface area than the rate of fluid flux in other capillary beds and, when multiplied by the total nephron population of about 2 million, yields a remarkably high filtration rate of about 180 liters per day.

The process of glomerular filtration, as with fluid movement across other capillary beds, derives its driving force from the hydraulic pressure originating in the pumping action of the heart. The actual rate of filtration is proportional to the net ultrafiltration pressure ($\bar{P}_{UF}$) existing across the capillary wall. This in turn is determined by the balance of hydraulic (P) and oncotic (Π) pressures (so-called Starling forces) that act between the glomerular capillary lumen and the surrounding tubule (Bowman's space). The ultrafiltration coefficient (K_f), a proportionality constant which relates the pressure gradient to the rate of fluid flux (i.e., the filtration rate), depends on both the intrinsic water permeability properties of the capillary wall (hydraulic permeability, k), and the available surface area (A). Thus,

Glomerular filtration is driven by hydraulic pressure. GFR depends on the balance of hydraulic and oncotic pressures between capillary and tubule.

$$
\begin{aligned}
SNGFR &= K_f \times \bar{P}_{UF} \\
&= K_f \left[(\bar{P}_{GC} - P_T) - (\bar{\Pi}_{GC} - \Pi_T) \right] \qquad (1) \\
&= k\,A\,(\overline{\Delta P} - \overline{\Delta \Pi})
\end{aligned}
$$

where the subscripts GC and T refer to glomerular capillary and tubule (i.e., Bowman's capsule) lumen, respectively, and the overbar indicates mean values.

Tubule fluid protein concentration is minimal and tubule fluid oncotic pressure is essentially zero.

The process of filtration yields a nearly ideal ultrafiltrate of plasma. Hence tubule fluid protein concentration is minimal, and the oncotic pressure (resulting from the colloidal properties of macromolecules) within the urinary space, Π_T, is essentially zero. Alterations in *plasma* protein concentrations exert significant effects on SNGFR, as evidenced in many patients by clinical observations. In those with marked hyperproteinemia, as in multiple myeloma, the elevated plasma oncotic pressure (high $\overline{\Pi}_{GC}$) contributes to a reduced GFR. Similar effects are seen with changes in $\overline{\Delta P}$: ureteral or intratubular obstruction, which raises P_T, lowers the net hydraulic force favoring filtration, and contributes to a fall in GFR.

Glomerular capillary hydraulic pressure is nearly constant and always higher than capillary oncotic pressure, which rises along the length of the capillary.

Since approximately 20 percent of the plasma water entering the glomerulus appears as filtrate, but only minimal quantities of plasma proteins are lost, the protein concentration (and Π_{GC}) is not constant, but rises along the length of the glomerular capillaries. A more detailed analysis of the forces governing filtration can be derived from a model which envisages an idealized glomerulus consisting of a single tube through which plasma enters at an initial flow rate (Q_A). Capillary oncotic pressure at the afferent end (Π_A) equals systemic plasma oncotic pressure, and the initial driving force for filtration is relatively high. However, as plasma water is filtered, the capillary oncotic pressure rises and the net filtration pressure declines. Direct measurements in various species indicate that $\overline{\Delta P}$ is approximately 35 mm Hg and is nearly constant along the length of the glomerular capillary, while Π_{GC} increases from about 20 mm Hg at the afferent end to 35 mm Hg at the efferent end (Fig. 1–11, left panel). Thus the net pressure gradient (P_{UF}) favors filtration throughout the length of the glomerular capillaries.

Factors contributing to high SNGFR:
- *Increased $\overline{\Delta P}$ (hypertension)*
- *Reduced plasma protein concentration (malnutrition)*
- *Increased glomerular plasma flow rate (anemia, pregnancy)*
- *Increased value of K_f (theoretical)*

This analysis provides an explanation for an important clinical observation: GFR tends to vary in parallel with RPF. Equation (1) describing the forces governing SNGFR does not include a specific term for RPF. But RPF is implicitly taken into account because the "profile" of Π_{GC} from the afferent to the efferent end of the capillary varies with Q_A (Fig. 1–11). With very high plasma flow, and a rapid transit time, a small fraction of the plasma will be filtered; thus Π_{GC} will not increase a great deal, $\overline{\Delta\Pi}$ will be lower, and the net driving force for filtration will be higher. Conversely, at low values for Q_A, Π_{GC} rises more rapidly, and overall filtration will be reduced. The direct effect of Q_A on SNGFR is not linear, however, so that extrapolations to clinical circumstances can be only approximate.

Factors contributing to low SNGFR:
- *Reduced $\overline{\Delta P}$ (hypotension, nephron obstruction)*
- *Increased plasma protein concentration (hyperglobulinemia)*
- *Reduced glomerular (renal) plasma flow rate (shock, dehydration)*
- *Reduced value of K_f (glomerulonephritis, vasoactive agents)*

One further level of sophistication is also needed in this discussion of the determinants of glomerular filtration rate. The value for $\overline{P}_{GC}$ is not related in a simple manner to mean arterial blood pressure. It depends in part on the resistance to flow provided by the afferent and efferent arterioles, and as discussed above, resistance is altered by intrinsic vascular tone, neural stimulation, and vasoactive hormones. Increases in efferent arteriolar resistance tend to *raise* pressure *upstream* in the glomerular capillary, thereby promoting glomerular filtration. Thus, it is the *balance* of afferent and efferent resistances that determines $\overline{\Delta P}$, whereas it is the *sum* of the two (i.e., total renal vascular resistance) that regulates Q_A.

The action of angiotensin II on glomerular hemodynamics provides a useful example of these principles. Infusion of pressor doses of AII

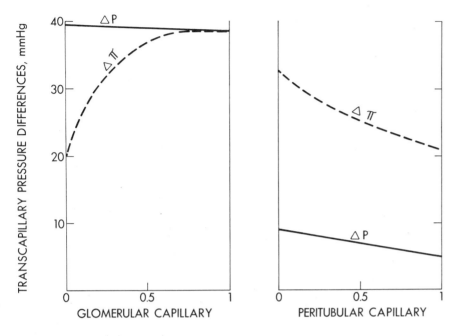

Figure 1–11. Diagram representing the oncotic and hydraulic pressure gradients governing fluid movement across glomerular and peritubular capillaries. In the glomerular capillaries the hydraulic pressure gradient (ΔP) is high and relatively constant; the oncotic pressure gradient opposing filtration ($\Delta\Pi$) is lower but rises along the length of the capillary as protein-free fluid is filtered. Nevertheless, the net ultrafiltration pressure ($\Delta P - \Delta\Pi$) always favors filtration. In peritubular capillaries ΔP is low because of high efferent arteriolar resistance. The high value for $\Delta\Pi$ produces a net force favoring fluid reabsorption. (From Brenner, B. M., and Rector, F. C., Jr., eds.: The Kidney, 3rd Edition. W. B. Saunders Co., Philadelphia, 1986, with permission.)

produces a substantial decline in Q_A, but much less of a reduction in SNGFR. The fact that SNGFR is sustained despite the fall in Q_A results from an increase in $\overline{\Delta P}$, a consequence of a rise in blood pressure and a relatively greater increase in efferent than afferent arteriolar resistance. A similar preferential vasoconstrictor effect on the efferent arteriole has been demonstrated for norepinephrine as well. These properties contribute to the *autoregulation* of GFR when renal perfusion pressure and RBF are reduced.

Glomerular capillary hydraulic pressure is determined by arterial blood pressure and by the varying vascular tone of the renal arterioles.

The ultrafiltration coefficient, K_f, is a dynamically modulated variable which contributes importantly to the control of SNGFR. Contained between glomerular capillaries are supporting *mesangial cells*, which serve a variety of functions including phagocytosis and catabolism of trapped immunoglobulins. In addition, mesangial cells contain intracellular *myofilaments* which contract in response to circulating vasoconstrictors, thereby reducing the surface area (A) available for filtration. Since K_f is proportional to A, reduction of surface area is an important additional mechanism by which renal vasoactive substances influence SNGFR. Indeed, experimental findings indicate that

Specialized mesangial cells between glomerular capillaries act to reduce capillary wall surface area in response to vasoconstrictors.

a decline in K_f is a consistent effect of many vasoactive agents. In a number of experimental and clinicopathologic conditions in which there is selective damage to glomerular capillaries (i.e., glomerulonephritis), the associated decline in K_f results from reduced surface area as well as direct damage to the glomerular capillary wall (causing reduced hydraulic conductivity).

GFR is affected by the rate of fluid delivery to the macula densa (tubuloglomerular feedback).

In addition to the influence of renal nerves and circulating and intrarenal hormones on GFR, the rate of fluid delivery to the macula densa region of the early distal tubule also regulates glomerular dynamics, so-called *tubuloglomerular feedback.* High distal tubule fluid flows and salt delivery rates produce a fall in SNGFR, largely related to increases in afferent and efferent arteriolar resistance and a decline in K_f. The precise effector mechanism is uncertain, but the close anatomic proximity of macula densa, mesangium, and afferent and efferent arterioles (Fig. 1–5) suggests a single process, perhaps related to AII-induced contraction of mesangial cells, which can reduce the caliber of attached arterioles and glomerular capillaries. The importance of tubuloglomerular feedback is most apparent in pathologic states where proximal tubule fluid reabsorption is impaired. If the high distal delivery rate did not reflexly reduce GFR, fluid transport mechanisms in the distal tubule would be overwhelmed, and excessive urinary fluid and electrolyte losses would ensue.

Glomerular capillary walls possess size-selective and charge-selective barriers to filtration.

Glomerular Barriers to Macromolecules. Despite the extremely high permeability of the glomerular capillary wall to water (~ 180 liters/day), plasma proteins are normally almost entirely excluded from the urinary space. Macromolecules in the size range below 20 Å molecular radius (e.g., inulin) are freely filtered, whereas the permeability of the capillary wall approaches zero as molecular radius increases toward 40 Å (Fig. 1–12). This size selectivity is consistent with the presence within the membrane of *"pores"* of specific dimensions and configuration limiting the passage of large solutes. Within the

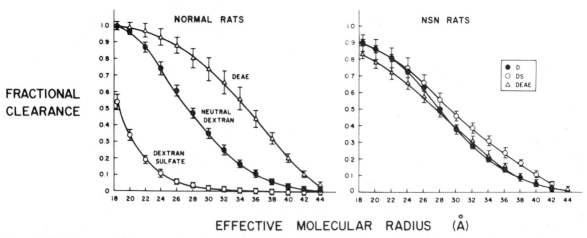

Figure 1–12. Fractional clearance of cationic (DEAE) dextran, neutral dextran (D), and anionic dextran sulfate (DS) in normal rats (left panel) and rats with proteinuria from experimental nephrotoxic serum nephritis (NSN) (right panel). The normal charge discrimination of the glomerular capillary wall is lost in NSN. (From Bohrer, M. P., et al.: Permselectivity of the glomerular capillary wall: facilitated filtration of circulating polycations. J. Clin. Invest. 61:72–78, 1978, with permission of The American Society for Clinical Investigation.)

glomerular capillary wall there exists also a *charge-selective barrier* to filtration: negatively charged macromolecules are impeded and positively charged ones facilitated in their transit across the capillary wall, compared with neutral compounds of the same size (Fig. 1–12, left panel). This property derives from the presence within the glomerular capillary wall of *fixed negative charges*, in part related to sialic acid residues within structural glycoproteins (Fig. 1–10). Such fixed negative charges are found in all regions of the capillary wall, including the surface coat of epithelial cell foot processes and the slit diaphragms which lie between adjacent pedicels. It is likely that the area closest to the endothelial surface serves as the primary, but not the sole barrier to the transit of anionic macromolecules.

The presence of proteinuria, a hallmark of renal disease, can be understood in terms of the charge- and size-selective properties of the glomerular wall. In an animal model of proteinuria (nephrotoxic serum nephritis, NSN) the charge selectivity of the glomerular wall is largely abolished (Fig. 1–12, right panel). Similarly, in human minimal-change nephropathy, where no gross structural damage is evident, proteinuria results almost exclusively from loss of fixed negative charges. In other disorders with prominent disruption of the glomerular architecture (e.g., lupus nephritis, advanced diabetic nephropathy) there is both an impaired charge selectivity and the presence of an abnormal number of pores of large size, the latter contributing to the enhanced "leakage" of large macromolecules from plasma.

THE CORTICAL PERITUBULAR MICROCIRCULATION

Of the 180 liters of glomerular filtrate produced daily, less than 1 percent is excreted as urine. The remainder is returned to the circulation in a two-stage process that involves translocation of fluid and solute across the tubule epithelium into the renal interstitium, and then uptake into the peritubular capillary blood. *Transepithelial* transport from tubule lumen to renal interstitium is discussed in detail in Chapter 2. The flux of fluid across the capillary wall proceeds by bulk flow, governed by the same interplay of hydraulic and oncotic forces (Starling forces) that governs glomerular filtration. Approximately two thirds of tubule fluid reabsorption occurs in the convoluted and straight portions of the proximal tubule, and it is in this region that the cortical peritubular circulation exerts its major influence on fluid reabsorption.

It is not possible to identify either the transepithelial (active) or the transcapillary (passive) transport step as the "rate limiting" process in the reabsorption of ultrafiltrate. Clearly, drugs that poison the metabolic machinery of tubule cells cause a profound impairment in the rate of fluid reabsorption. However, maneuvers which markedly lessen the transcapillary (Starling) driving force for uptake of reabsorbate into the cortical peritubular capillaries will also depress net fluid reabsorption. Under these circumstances cellular active transport continues to deliver luminal fluid to the cortical interstitium. As fluid accumulates, a second mechanism for fluid removal from the interstitium gains increasing importance. Despite the presence of apical tight junctions, the space between adjacent renal proximal tubule epithelial

Reabsorption of glomerular filtrate involves active transport across tubule epithelium and passive uptake across cortical peritubular capillary walls.

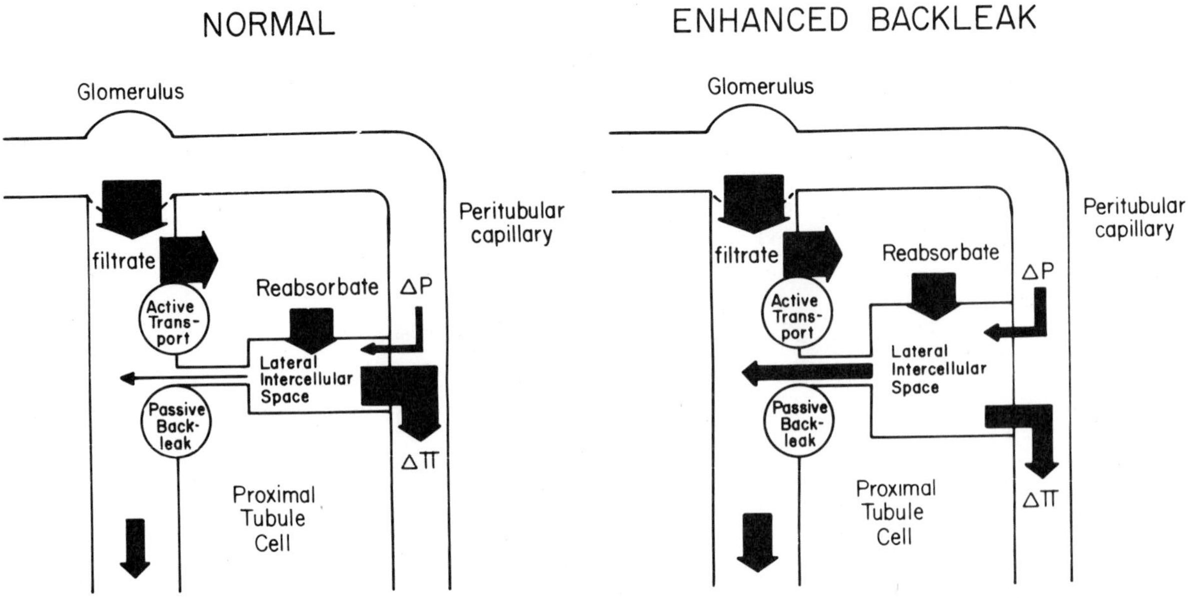

Figure 1–13. Regulation of fluid uptake into peritubular capillaries. Left panel: under normal conditions filtrate is absorbed into proximal tubule cells, actively transported into lateral intercellular spaces, and taken up into peritubular capillaries by the influence of Starling forces. Right panel: when the driving force for reabsorption is lessened (increased ΔP, reduced $\Delta \Pi$), fluid that accumulates in lateral intercellular spaces returns to the tubule lumen by passive backleak. (Adapted from Humes, H. D., et al.: The kidney in congestive heart failure. *In* Brenner, B. M., and Stein, J. H., eds.: Contemporary Issues in Nephrology, Vol. 1: Sodium and Water Homeostasis. Churchill Livingstone, New York, 1978, with permission.)

cells is not wholly impermeable to fluid. When the transcapillary driving force is reduced, *backleak* occurs as interstitial fluid returns to the tubule lumen (Fig. 1–13). Thus, even though active transport proceeds as usual, alterations in peritubular capillary Starling forces may exert an important regulatory influence on the overall rate of tubule fluid reabsorption. Indeed, in certain animal models, the effect of Starling forces on proximal fluid reabsorption is so profound that the overall process of fluid reabsorption can be modelled as if transcapillary exchange were the only regulatory mechanism involved. Nevertheless, as discussed in Chapter 2, the precise *composition* of the reabsorbed fluid is determined by the selective transport of individual solutes across the renal epithelial cells. In this fashion the renal tubule cell serves not simply as a conduit for the bulk reabsorption of tubule fluid, but rather as a crucial regulator of body fluid composition.

Alterations in capillary Starling forces affect the rate of reabsorption, but the composition of the reabsorbed fluid is determined by selective transport across tubule epithelium.

Having indicated how peritubular capillary Starling forces may affect tubule transport functions, it is important to outline the anatomic and physiologic features of this microcirculation that facilitate the interplay of capillary and tubule events. Since the major portion of tubule fluid reabsorption occurs in the convoluted and straight portions of the proximal tubule, it is understandable that the cortical peritubular capillary network lies in close apposition to these nephron segments (Fig. 1–2). Indeed the capillary vessels which surround the tubule convolutions are composed of a single layer of fenestrated endothelial cells, surrounded only by a thin basement membrane, thus facilitating the rapid movement of fluid over a short distance from interstitium to capillary lumen. These peritubular vessels, as well as those perfusing other tubule structures (i.e., distal convoluted tubules, loops of Henle, and collecting ducts contained within the medullary rays) all derive from glomerular efferent arterioles. This *portal circulation* is distinctive in that the efferent arteriole that connects the glomerular and peritubular circulations contributes a significant resistance to blood flow. The result is a low hydraulic pressure (10 to 15 mm Hg) at the beginning of the peritubular capillary network (Fig. 1–11, right panel), and a similar low value for $\overline{\Delta P}$ of 5 to 8 mm Hg. Glomerular filtration also increases the oncotic pressure within the peritubular capillaries by raising the concentration of proteins within the efferent plasma. Since no significant reabsorption occurs along the thicker-walled efferent arteriole itself, the plasma delivered to the peritubular microcirculation also has a high oncotic pressure, approximately 35 mm Hg. Interstitial oncotic pressure is estimated at 3 to 6 mm Hg, yielding values for $\overline{\Delta\Pi}$ of about 30 mm Hg. The net pressure gradient $(\overline{\Delta\Pi} - \overline{\Delta P})$ is therefore approximately 20 to 25 mm Hg. Just as the pressure gradient ($\Delta P - \Delta\Pi$) declines along the glomerular capillaries, so ($\Delta\Pi - \Delta P$) declines along the peritubular capillary network as reabsorbed fluid dilutes the plasma proteins, but the net driving force at the distal end is still about 10 to 15 mm Hg. The reabsorptive process, therefore, never reaches equilibrium and always favors fluid uptake into the peritubular capillaries. Reabsorption is relatively insensitive to alterations in local capillary plasma flow rate. Values for the peritubular capillary ultrafiltration coefficient are similar to those for the glomerular capillary wall, owing primarily to the very large surface area of this highly branched microvasculature which further facilitates the process of proximal tubule fluid reabsorption.

Cortical peritubular capillary oncotic pressure is high while interstitial oncotic pressure is low. Hydraulic pressure in these capillaries is always lower than oncotic pressure, promoting fluid reabsorption.

To understand how physiologic perturbations of the organism influence the operation of the cortical peritubular vasculature, consider the effects of a decline in intravascular volume such as may be induced by hemorrhage. As renal perfusion pressure declines, systemic and local renal compensatory mechanisms, including increased renal nerve traffic and circulating angiotensin II concentrations, tend to minimize the fall in GFR, primarily by augmenting efferent arteriolar resistance disproportionately to afferent resistance. Glomerular plasma flow is reduced more than GFR, leading to a rise in *filtration fraction* (GFR/RPF). The plasma exiting the efferent vasculature thus has an exaggerated rise in oncotic pressure and a reduced hydraulic pressure, precisely the conditions which enhance reabsorption of fluid from the proximal tubule (Fig. 1–13). Experimental and clinical measurements under conditions of renal hypoperfusion demonstrate the predicted rise in the fraction of glomerular filtrate reabsorbed in the proximal tubule. Conversely, under conditions in which GFR is enhanced and the glomerular resistance vessels are relatively relaxed (e.g., intravascular volume expansion), the observed decline in fractional proximal reabsorption can again be explained simply by the changes in postglomerular capillary hydraulic and oncotic pressure gradients.

Thus, alterations in glomerular dynamics have an important regulatory influence on the cortical peritubular capillary circulation. The same glomerular mechanisms which preserve GFR when renal perfusion is impaired mitigate the excessive urinary loss of essential body fluids by augmenting the proportion of filtered water and solutes

Reabsorption is regulated in part by alterations in GFR and in glomerular arteriolar resistance.

reabsorbed in the proximal nephron. This protective mechanism, coupled with additional fluid and sodium reabsorptive processes in the loop of Henle, distal tubule, and collecting duct, is fundamental to the preservation of intravascular volume and renal perfusion when threatened by hemorrhage, congestive heart failure, liver disease, or extrarenal losses of fluid.

The close relationship between glomerular and peritubular circulations in regulating tubule fluid suggests that each nephron and its vasculature function as an isolated, independent unit. In fact, this interpretation is most nearly correct only for superficial cortical glomeruli. Here the capillary bed that perfuses the proximal and distal convoluted tubules is entirely derived from the efferent arteriole of the parent glomerulus (Fig. 1–2). In the midcortex, efferent arterioles of many different glomeruli provide perfusion to each convoluted tubule. Other efferent arterioles extend to the *medullary rays* to perfuse portions of nephrons (i.e., proximal straight tubule, thick ascending limb of Henle's loop, collecting duct) derived from glomeruli lying in more superficial regions of the cortex. In the inner cortex, some efferent arterioles contribute the vascular supply to nearby proximal tubules of other nephrons, whereas others provide circulation to medullary structures.

THE MEDULLARY MICROCIRCULATION

The vascular supply to the medulla is derived from the efferent arterioles of glomeruli lying within the inner cortex (Fig. 1–2). As many as 10 such efferent vessels descend in parallel into the outer medulla as a *vascular bundle*, there giving rise to a dense capillary network. This microvasculature provides perfusion to all of the tubule structures contained within the *outer medulla:* proximal straight tubule segments, thin descending and thick ascending limbs of Henle's loop, and collecting ducts. Drainage of the capillary vessels is by veins which ascend to the inner cortex among the tubules and not within the vascular bundles themselves.

Only a portion of the vessels within vascular bundles of the outer medulla give rise to capillaries which perfuse structures within this region. Vessels located in the center of vascular bundles descend directly to the *inner medulla* in a straight, unbranching fashion (hence the term *vasa recta*) and give rise to a simple capillary network that surrounds the deep medullary tubule structures—thin descending and ascending limbs, and collecting ducts. The draining vessels (ascending vasa recta) are also straight and unbranching. They lie alongside the descending vasa recta within the vascular bundles as they course toward larger venous structures at the *corticomedullary junction.* Close anatomic proximity and precise alignment of ascending and descending vessels are essential for the efficient operation of the renal concentrating mechanism.

Like the cortical peritubular circulations, the medullary microvasculature serves to provide metabolic substrates to tubule structures and to remove waste products. In addition, an important fraction of tubule fluid reabsorption (20 to 30 percent) occurs within the renal medulla. Hence, fluid transported from tubule lumen to the medullary interstitium by active transport or passive mechanisms must be efficiently returned to the blood to permit maintenance of overall fluid balance. Starling forces operating across the medullary peritubular vessels regulate fluid reabsorption from the medullary interstitium, just as they modulate fluid uptake into the cortical vasculature.

A gradient of increasing interstitial solute concentration exists from the corticomedullary junction to the papillary tip, an essential component of the system for excreting urine of high osmolality (Fig. 1–14). This solute gradient has no direct influence on the pressure gradients that exist between the interstitium and the medullary vessels, because the small solutes that account for the axial concentration gradient (primarily sodium, chloride, and urea) are freely diffusible across the capillary wall. However, the descending vasa recta are essentially impermeable to proteins, and the high protein concentration of the entering plasma produces an effective oncotic pressure gradient. The value for $\Delta\Pi$ in descending vasa recta (about 35 mm Hg) is similar to values within cortical efferent arterioles, from which the vasa recta are derived. The balance of hydraulic pressures between vessel lumen (~10 mm Hg) and interstitium (estimated at 3 to 6 mm Hg) yields values for the net pressure gradient of approximately 20 mm Hg in favor of capillary fluid uptake, a significant gradient facilitating the rapid reabsorption of interstitial fluid into the medullary vessels.

The medullary capillary net pressure gradient, like that in the cortex, facilitates tubule fluid reabsorption into vessels.

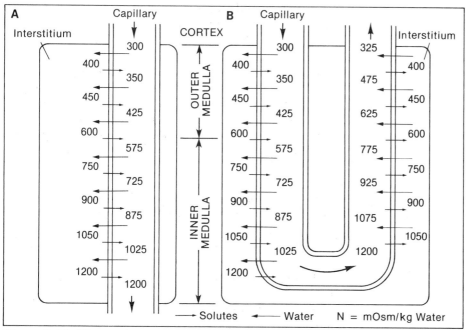

Figure 1–14. The renal countercurrent exchange system. Blood entering the loop at a concentration of 300 mOsm/liter encounters increasing interstitial solute concentrations, causing water to diffuse out of the capillary and solutes to diffuse in. In the ascending limb the process is reversed, so that the exiting plasma is only slightly concentrated (325 mOsm/liter), and the medullary solute gradient is not disturbed. (Illustration by Albert Miller; from Brenner, B. M., and Beeuwkes, R., III: The renal circulations. Hosp. Prac. 13:35–46, 1978, with permission.)

Increasing interstitial solute concentrations along the loop of Henle draw water from the tubule by osmosis. The hairpin structure of the medullary microcirculation facilitates removal of this fluid to prevent dilution of the interstitial solute gradient.

The existence of the corticomedullary interstitial solute gradient introduces major constraints on medullary hemodynamics which are reflected in certain unique features of the medullary microcirculation. As detailed in Chapter 3, the ability to elaborate a concentrated urine requires that water be abstracted from the collecting duct lumen by the osmotic effect of the hyperosmotic medullary interstitium. To prevent the dilution of this gradient by the reabsorbed water, the local circulation must function efficiently to remove fluid from the medullary interstitium. The numbers of ascending vasa recta are significantly greater than those of descending vasa recta, providing the capacity to accommodate the volume of fluid added to the medullary plasma. As discussed earlier, the inner medullary blood flow rate of 30 to 60 ml/100 gm/min, is not dissimilar from that of other well-perfused tissues. If the hyperosmolar inner medulla were perfused at this rate by blood of normal osmolality, the high medullary solute concentration would be rapidly abolished, and the concentrating mechanism would cease to function. A unique structural specialization of the medullary microcirculations permits the apparently conflicting requirement to be met. By arranging ascending and descending vessels adjacent and in parallel, a *countercurrent exchange* mechanism is created in which perfusion by isosmolar blood does not disrupt the medullary hyperosmolality created by tubule active transport processes.

The principle of countercurrent exchange.

The principle of a countercurrent exchanger can be described simply by analogy to the flow of water through a pipe which is heated by a flame. When the pipe is straight and the flame is placed at its center, fluid flowing through it will rapidly carry away the heat; the temperature of the outgoing fluid will be higher than that which enters, but the temperature adjacent to the flame is only modestly elevated because of the cooling effect of the incoming fluid. If the pipe is bent into a tight hairpin loop so that there is contact between the two limbs and the pipe is heated at its tip, a different situation develops. The warm departing fluid heats the cooler incoming fluid and will itself be cooled almost to the temperature at the inlet. However, the temperature at the heated tip will be higher than when the pipe is straight. Countercurrent flow, combined with efficient heat transfer, permits the flow of cool fluid into the system without causing dissipation of the heat contained within the loop.

The concentration gradient within the renal medulla and the countercurrent flow of blood in the medullary vascular bundles provide nature's counterpart to this model. Ascending and descending vasa recta approach osmotic equilibrium because of their proximity and their high solute and water permeability. Multiple vessels contained within the medullary vascular bundles have a much larger cross-sectional area than the efferent arterioles from which they were derived. *Flow velocity* within the loop is correspondingly reduced, so that the transit time of erythrocytes through the inner medulla is approximately 30–40 sec, or about 20 times slower than the transit time in the renal cortical peritubular microvasculature. The net result of this slow transit time is to promote osmotic equilibrium between ascending and descending vessels.

As blood enters the hyperosmolar inner medulla, solutes diffuse along concentration gradients from the renal interstitium into the more dilute plasma of the descending vasa recta, while water moves in the opposite direction along its osmotic gradient (Fig. 1–14). A progressive rise in the osmolality of the descending blood ensues, reaching its maximum at the hairpin turn. As blood ascends again, the opposite processes occur; interstitial water derived from reabsorption across medullary nephron segments is taken up in the ascending vasa recta, diluting the plasma to nearly the osmolality of the entering blood. This arrangement permits relatively normal rates of blood flow to the medulla without dissipating interstitial hyperosmotic gradients.

MEASUREMENT OF RENAL BLOOD FLOW

The measurement of renal blood flow is possible under both experimental and clinical circumstances. The most common method employs the *Fick principle* and the extraction of *para-aminohippuric acid (PAH)*. PAH is used because it is removed from the renal plasma with high efficiency and is neither metabolized nor synthesized within the kidney. The quantity of PAH removed from the plasma and delivered into the urine, $U_{PAH}V$ (where U_{PAH} = urine PAH concentration and V = urine flow rate), equals the amount extracted by the kidney. According to the Fick principle this quantity is given by the arteriovenous PAH concentration difference ($A_{PAH} - V_{PAH}$) multiplied by renal *plasma* flow rate (RPF), since PAH is present only in the plasma portion of blood. Thus,

Blood flow through an organ can be determined by measuring the amount of a substance removed from each unit quantity of blood as it passes through the organ and the total amount of the substance removed over a period of time (the Fick principle).

$$U_{PAH}V = RPF \times (A_{PAH} - V_{PAH}) \tag{2}$$

Rearranging yields:

$$RPF = \frac{U_{PAH}V}{A_{PAH} - V_{PAH}} \tag{3}$$

Renal blood flow can therefore be calculated:

$$RBF = RPF \times (1 - Hct) \tag{4}$$

where hematocrit (Hct) is expressed in fractional terms. About 90 percent of PAH is extracted in a single pass across the renal vasculature in normal humans when plasma PAH concentration is allowed to range from 1 to 6 mg/dl. Under these circumstances the renal venous PAH concentration is low, and neglecting this term (J_{PAH}) introduces an error of only about 10 percent in the calculation of RPF, an accuracy which is adequate for most clinical studies. Thus, Equation (3) simplifies to:

$$RPF = \frac{U_{PAH}V}{A_{PAH}} \tag{5}$$

However, in renal diseases and certain pathophysiologic states, extraction of PAH can be reduced, and the measurement of renal venous PAH concentration becomes necessary for accurate determination of PAH clearance.

Other techniques for the measurement of RBF, particularly the *insert gas (xenon) washout technique,* provide evidence that intrarenal perfusion is *heterogeneous,* both between the cortex and medulla, and within each region. In general, blood flow is highest in the outer cortex and declines progressively toward the inner medulla. It is uncertain whether the intracortical gradient reflects differences in plasma flow per glomerulus (Q_A) or in the density of glomeruli. A variety of physiologic perturbations (e.g., infusion of angiotensin II, neural stimulation, sodium depletion, and disease states such as shock or severe liver disease) produce preferential reduction of flow to outer cortical regions, so-called "intrarenal shunting." The possible role of changes in the intracortical distribution of blood flow in modulating sodium excretion, perhaps by shifting blood flow to more salt-avid juxtamedullary nephrons, remains controversial.

REFERENCES

General

Brenner, B. M., and Rector, F. C., Jr., eds.: The Kidney, 3rd Edition. W. B. Saunders Co., Philadelphia, 1986.
  A standard reference text on kidney physiology and clinical nephrology. The chapters dealing with anatomy of the kidney, the renal circulations, renal metabolism, glomerular filtration, control of extracellular fluid volume, renal vasoactive hormones, and urine concentration and dilution are particularly valuable for the beginning and intermediate student.

Brenner, B. M., and Beeuwkes, R., III: The renal circulations. Hosp. Prac. 13:35–46, 1978.
  A well-illustrated summary of renal circulatory anatomy and physiology.

Orloff, J., and Berliner, R. W.: Handbook of Physiology, Section 8: Renal Physiology. American Physiological Society, Washington, D.C., 1973.
  A definitive, although somewhat dated, review.

Pitts, R. F.: Physiology of the Kidney and Body Fluids, 3rd Edition. Year Book Medical Publishers, Inc., Chicago, 1974.
  A classic introductory text on renal physiology, emphasizing the fundamental features of kidney function.

Anatomy

Barger, A. C., and Herd, J. A.: The renal circulation. N. Engl. J. Med. 284:482–490, 1971.
  A beautiful photographic essay of renal vascular anatomy.

Beeuwkes, R., III, and Bonventre, J. V.: Tubular organization and vascular-tubular relations in the dog kidney. Am. J. Physiol. 229:695–713, 1975.
  An important topographical study of the anatomy of the canine kidney.

Fawcett, D. W.: A Textbook of Histology, 11th Edition. W. B. Saunders Co., Philadelphia, 1986.
Heptinstall, R. H.: Pathology of the Kidney, 3rd Edition. Little, Brown and Company, Boston, 1983.
  These two textbooks contain chapters with readable and detailed descriptions of renal anatomy.

Regulation of Renal Vascular Tone

Autoregulation

Navar, L. E.: Renal autoregulation: perspectives from whole-kidney and single-nephron studies. Am. J. Physiol. 234:F357, 1978.
  A review of the hormonal, neural, and myogenic control of renal vascular tone.

Renin-Angiotensin-Aldosterone System

Reid, I. A., Morris, B. J., and Ganong, W. F.: The renin-angiotensin system. Ann Rev. Physiol. 40:377–410, 1978.
  A brief review of renin-angiotensin biochemistry and physiology.

Renal Nerves

DiBona, G. F.: The functions of the renal nerves. Rev. Physiol. Biochem. Pharmacol. 94:75–181, 1983.
The innervation of the kidney, and the influence of renal nerves on RBF, GFR, and sodium metabolism are the topics of this excellent review.

Prostaglandins

Levenson, D. J., Simmons, C. E., Jr., and Brenner, B. M.: Arachidonic acid metabolism, prostaglandins and the kidney. Am. J. Med. 72:354–374, 1982.
Detailed, current review of renal prostaglandins and their role in regulating hemodynamics and renal excretory functions.

Kallikrein-Kinins

Carretero, O. A., and Scicli, A. G.: The renal kallikrein-kinin system. Am. J. Physiol. 238:F246–F255, 1980.
The biochemistry, physiologic actions, and pathophysiologic roles of this hormone system are succinctly presented.

Atrial Peptides

Ballermann, B. J., and Brenner, B. M.: Biologically active atrial peptides. J. Clin. Invest. 76:2041–2048, 1985.
A comprehensive and current review of the renal and extrarenal actions of atrial peptides.

Mechanisms of Ultrafiltration

Baylis, C., and Brenner, B. M.: The physiologic determinants of glomerular ultrafiltration. Rev. Physiol. Biochem. Pharmacol. 80:1–46, 1978.
This article presents the theoretical and experimental data regarding the determinants of single nephron GFR.

Brenner, B. M., and Humes, H. D.: Mechanics of glomerular ultrafiltration. N. Engl. J. Med. 297:148–154, 1977.
An introduction to the processes governing glomerular filtration.

Dworkin, L. D., Ichikawa, I., and Brenner, B. M.: Humoral modulation of glomerular function. Am. J. Physiol. 244:F95–F104, 1983.
This review describes the effects of various hormones on renal vascular resistances, the ultrafiltration coefficient, and SNGFR.

Wright, F. S., and Briggs, J. P.: Feedback regulation of glomerular filtration rate. Am. J. Physiol. 233:F1–F7, 1977.
This editorial summarizes the data supporting the existence of feedback regulation of GFR, and describes the sensor and effector mechanisms that govern its operation.

Glomerular Filtration of Macromolecules

Brenner, B. M., Hostetter, T. H., and Humes, H. D.: Molecular basis of proteinuria of glomerular origin. N. Engl. J. Med. 198:826–833, 1978.
A brief exposition of the structural and biochemical properties of the glomerular barrier to the filtration of macromolecules.

Deen, W. M., Bridges, C. R., and Brenner, B. M.: Biophysical basis of glomerular permselectivity. Biophysical J. 71:1–10, 1983.
Recent comprehensive discussion of the biophysics of charge- and size-selectivity of the glomerular capillary wall.

Cortical Peritubular Microcirculations

Baylis, C.: Control of sodium reabsorption and its relation to renal hemodynamics. Sem. Nephrol. 3:180–195, 1983.
A readable summary of the role of Starling forces in the control of tubule sodium reabsorption.

Humes, H. D., Gottlieb, M. N., and Brenner, B. M.: The kidney in congestive heart failure. *In* Brenner, B. M., and Stein, J. H., eds.: Contemporary Issues in Nephrology, Vol. 1: Sodium and Water Homeostasis. Churchill Livingstone Inc., New York, 1978.
Discusses the role of peritubular factors in the sodium retention of heart failure.

Ichikawa, I., and Brenner, B. M.: Mechanism of inhibition of proximal tubule fluid reabsorption after exposure of the kidney to the physical effects of expansion of extracellular fluid volume. J. Clin. Invest. 64:1466–1474, 1979.
An experimental study demonstrating the influence of peritubular Starling forces on proximal tubule fluid reabsorption.

Medullary Microcirculation

Marsh, D. J., and Segel, L. A.: Analysis of countercurrent diffusion exchange in blood vessels of the renal medulla. Am. J. Physiol. 221:817–828, 1971.
A theoretical analysis of the countercurrent exchange mechanism.

Measurement of Renal Blood Flow

Brenner, B. M., Zatz, R., and Ichikawa, I.: The renal circulations. *In* Brenner, B. M., and Rector, F. C., Jr., eds.: The Kidney, 3rd Edition. W. B. Saunders Co., Philadelphia, 1986.
The various methods currently in use for measuring renal blood flow and intrarenal blood flow distribution are considered.

Transport Functions of the Renal Tubules

ANATOMY OF THE RENAL TUBULES
BASIC MECHANISMS OF TRANSPORT IN EPITHELIA
PROXIMAL TUBULE SEGMENTS
   First Phase of Proximal Reabsorption
   Second Phase of Proximal Reabsorption
   Capillary Uptake of Proximal Reabsorbate
   Secretion of Organic Ions
THIN LIMBS OF THE LOOP OF HENLE
DISTAL TUBULE SEGMENTS
COLLECTING TUBULE SEGMENTS
   NaCl Transport
   K^+ Transport
   H^+ and HCO_3^- Transport
   Water Transport
   Urea Transport
   Mineralocorticoid Hormone Control of Na^+, K^+, and H^+ Transport
   Antidiuretic Hormone Control of Water Transport
URINE CONCENTRATION AND DILUTION

Approximately 180 liters of protein-free fluid are produced by glomerular ultrafiltration each day (Table 2–1). This fluid contains sodium and its attendant anions (chloride, bicarbonate, phosphate) as the principal osmotic solutes, plus smaller amounts of other essential electrolytes and organic solutes, as well as metabolic waste products.

Table 2–1. AVERAGE EXCRETION VALUES FOR SUBSTANCES FILTERED

Substance (units)	Amount Filtered	Amount Excreted	Percent Reabsorbed
Water (liter)	180	0.5–3.0	98–99
Sodium (mEq)	25,000	50–200	99+
Chloride (mEq)	19,500	50–200	99+
Bicarbonate (mEq)	4,500	0	100
Potassium (mEq)	720	40–120	80–95
Glucose (gm)	180	0	100
Urea (gm)	56	28	50

Approximately 1 to 2 percent of the water, less than 1 percent of the filtered sodium, and variable amounts of the other solutes are excreted in the final urine. During the course of processing this large quantity of fluid and solutes, the renal tubules homeostatically control the volume, osmolality, composition, and acidity of the intra- and extracellular fluid compartments with great precision. Essential nutrients (sugars, Krebs cycle intermediates, amino acids) are avidly conserved, while metabolic waste products are efficiently removed or cleared from the body.

ANATOMY OF THE RENAL TUBULES

Each human kidney contains over one million nephrons. The nephron begins in the renal cortex with the renal corpuscles, which consist of an arterial capillary tuft or glomerulus and a blind expansion of the renal tubule, Bowman's capsule. Glomeruli are distinguished within the kidney by their relative positions in the renal cortex: superficial, midcortical, and juxtamedullary renal glomeruli (Figs. 2–1 and 2–2). Similarly, nephrons are classified according to the position of their glomeruli: superficial, midcortical, and juxtamedullary nephrons. Superficial glomeruli have efferent arterioles which ascend to the surface of the renal cortex. Juxtamedullary glomeruli have efferent arterioles which give rise to the descending vasa recta and thus provide the blood supply for the renal medulla. In the rabbit, 28 percent of the glomeruli are superficial and 9 percent are juxtamedullary. The remaining 63 percent are midcortical.

The two tubule segments of the nephron—the proximal tubule system and the distal tubule system—act in concert to maintain solute and water balance.

The tubule portion of the nephron can be divided into two groups of tubule segments: the *proximal tubule system* and the *distal tubule system* (Fig. 2–2). Within each of these nephron segments the tubules are lined with epithelial cells of a single type, although the cell types differ from one segment to another. The proximal tubule system is 10 to 12 mm in length. Its primary function is to reabsorb essential nutrients, filtered salts, and water, and to secrete unessential waste products. The distal tubule system is composed of the thick ascending limb and the true distal tubule. These two segments are about 3 to 4 mm in length. Their main function is to dilute the tubule fluid by reabsorbing sodium in excess of water. The thin limbs of the loop of Henle and the distal tubule system act together with the variable water and urea permeability of the collecting tubule system to form either a dilute or a concentrated urine. These tubule segments maintain water balance.

Nephrons have also been divided into two types according to the length of their loops of Henle: short- and long-looped nephrons. Short-looped nephrons form the bend of Henle within the outer medulla. Long-looped nephrons penetrate into the inner medulla. In general, nephrons with superficial glomeruli have short loops and nephrons with juxtamedullary glomeruli have long loops. Nephrons with midcortical glomeruli have both long and short loops. The ratio of short- to long-looped nephrons varies from species to species. Although absence of long loops impairs concentrating ability, a preponderance of long loops does not enhance the ability of the kidney to generate a

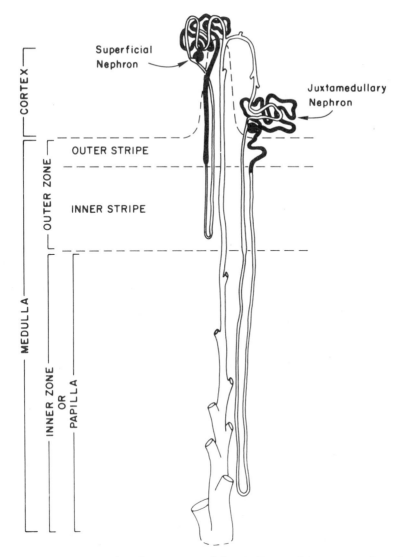

Figure 2–1. Two principal nephron types and their collecting duct systems. Superficial nephrons have their glomeruli near the surface of the kidney and do not possess long loops of Henle. Juxtamedullary nephrons have their glomeruli at the corticomedullary junction. Glomeruli and proximal tubules are in solid black. The remaining nephron is in white.

concentrated urine. It is the length of the long loops rather than their number that is important to urine concentration.

Anywhere from five to ten nephrons drain into a single cortical *collecting duct* (Fig. 2–2). In the inner medulla about eight collecting ducts fuse, so that the final collecting duct drains around 3,000 nephrons. One of the more striking characteristics of the collecting tubule system is its lining by mixed rather than homogeneous cell types. Thus the connecting tubule (segment 10 in Fig. 2–2), which is composed of two cell types, is included in the collecting rather than the distal tubule system, despite the fact that there are as many connecting tubules as there are nephrons. That the cell types differ is probably related to the diverse function of the collecting tubule system in the ultimate, fine control of all solute excretion.

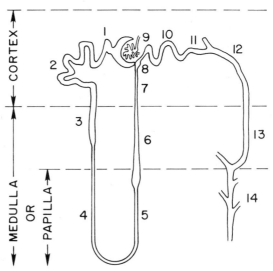

Figure 2–2. Individual tubule segments, schematically represented. The proximal nephron contains the proximal tubule system (1–3) and the thin limbs (4, 5). The distal nephron contains the distal tubule system (6–9) and the collecting tubule system (10–14).

(1) initial proximal convoluted tubule, S1; (2) late proximal convoluted tubule and early proximal straight tubule, S2; (3) late proximal straight tubule, S3; (4) thin descending limb of Henle's loop; (5) thin ascending limb of Henle's loop; (6) medullary thick ascending limb of Henle's loop; (7) cortical thick ascending limb of Henle's loop; (8) macula densa; (9) distal convoluted tubule; (10) connecting tubule; (11) initial collecting tubule; (12) cortical collecting tubule; (13) outer medullary collecting tubule; (14) papillary collecting tubule.

BASIC MECHANISMS OF TRANSPORT IN EPITHELIA

Epithelia, whether lining bags like the gallbladder or urinary bladder or tubes like the nephron or the intestine, have the unique capacity to transport solutes and water from one surface to another. Enabling epithelia to perform this vectoral transport is the polarization of the cell membrane into *apical and basolateral membranes* (Fig. 2–3). Because the apical membrane is both structurally and functionally different from the basolateral membrane, directional transport takes place. The structural polarization cannot be random; it must be consistently oriented in the same direction by the so-called *junctional complexes.* The best model of oriented epithelia in its sheet form is the current method of packaging a six-pack of beer. The epithelial cells (the beer cans) are held together by junctional complexes (the plastic mesh) and separated by lateral intercellular spaces (the areas between cans). The junctional complexes (the plastic mesh) also serve to separate the apical surface (tops of cans) from the basolateral surface (sides and bottoms of cans).

Generally the epithelial basolateral surface possesses the ubiquitous primary active transport mechanism, the *Na$^+$-K$^+$ ATPase pump system.* The apical surface generally possesses either diffusional or carrier-mediated mechanisms for Na$^+$ transport. The separation or polarization of these two types of transport mechanisms on these two separate membranes (which face different fluid compartments) enables

"Junctional complexes" provide the structural orientation of epithelia necessary for directional transport of solutes and water.

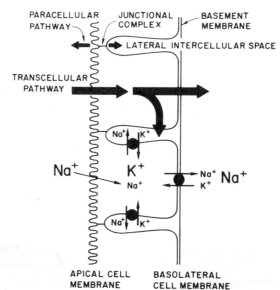

Figure 2–3. Schematic representation of proximal tubule cell. The transcellular transport pathway consists of apical and basolateral cell membranes. The paracellular transport pathway consists of junctional complexes and lateral intercellular spaces. Intracellular Na^+ concentration is maintained below and intracellular K^+ concentration is maintained above plasma by the Na^+-K^+ ATPase pump system.

transepithelial transport to occur. The basolateral membrane transport system actively pumps to maintain a low cellular Na^+ concentration. Extracellular Na^+, however, continues to be high. As a result, the Na^+ entry mechanisms located in the apical membrane allow Na^+ to move from its higher concentration in the luminal fluid to its lower concentration inside the cell. The Na^+-K^+ ATPase pump system senses the addition of Na^+ to the cell and is stimulated to increase its rate of pumping in order to return the cell Na^+ to its low level. The net effect of these two steps is transport of Na^+ from the apical fluid compartment to the basolateral fluid compartment.

The differences between apical and basolateral membrane properties account for the transepithelial transport of all solutes. Most transepithelial transport requires the expenditure of metabolic energy and thus requires solute transport to interact actively with the cell membranes. This active form of transepithelial transport is said to use the *transcellular pathway*. Alternatively, it is possible that the transepithelial transport pathway could bypass the cell and solutes and/or water might cross the epithelium by purely passive mechanisms. This type of transport is said to be paracellular. The *paracellular transport pathway* consists of the junctional complexes and the lateral intercellular spaces. If the junctional complexes are highly permeable to solutes, the paracellular pathway will act to dissipate any concentration gradient generated by active transcellular transport. In some cases this dissipation can be advantageous for epithelial function. Generally, epithelia whose principal role is the transport of large quantities of solute and water without the generation of significant concentration gradients, like the proximal nephron segments, have highly permeable junctional complexes. On the other hand, epithelia whose principal function is the generation of large solute concentration differences, like the collecting tubule system, have very low-permeability junctional complexes.

Transepithelial transport of solute follows either transcellular (active) or paracellular (passive) pathways.

PROXIMAL TUBULE SEGMENTS

The proximal nephron can be divided into three distinct tubule segments: the early proximal convoluted tubule or S1, the remaining cortical proximal tubule or S2, and the medullary proximal tubule S3. These segments differ from each other morphologically in that early segments have greater membrane surface area, enhanced numbers of mitochondria, and as might be expected, greater rates of solute reabsorption. Only recently has come sufficient understanding of the physiology of the proximal nephron to divide it into these distinct functional segments. Although all segments perform similar transport functions (except that the S2 segment predominates in organic anion and cation secretion), the quantitative properties of both the transcellular and the paracellular transport pathways vary inversely with the segment's distance from the glomerulus. In the early proximal convoluted tubule transcellular transport rates are rapid, but because the paracellular pathways are leakier, maximal solute gradients cannot be obtained. In the late proximal straight tubule the transcellular transport rates are slow, but because the paracellular pathways are tighter, maximal solute concentration gradients can be achieved. This arrangement of transcellular transporters and paracellular permeabilities along the proximal nephron enables the kidney to recover the bulk of the essential nutrients from the tubule fluid.

The proximal tubule segments reabsorb at least 60 percent of the glomerular ultrafiltrate. This process occurs without a measurable change in Na^+ concentration and only a slight fall (3 to 6 mOsm/kg) in tubule fluid osmolality. Thus, the proximal tubule reabsorbs at least 60 percent of the filtered water and Na^+ salts. The energy for virtually all of proximal reabsorption is derived from the Na^+-K^+ ATPase pump system located in the basolateral cell membrane.

Roughly 60 percent of the glomerular filtrate is reabsorbed in proximal tubule segments by an essentially isosmotic process.

The transport of solutes out of the proximal tubule is best described in two phases. As shown in Figure 2–4, in the early proximal tubule the tubule fluid (TF) to plasma (P) ratios of glucose, amino acids, and HCO_3^- decrease and the *electrical potential difference (PD)* is lumen-negative. This is the first phase of proximal reabsorption and it effects the preferential reabsorption of the esential nutrients, like neutral organic solutes and $NaHCO_3$. In the late proximal tubule the Cl^- concentration is elevated and the PD is lumen-positive. This is the second phase of proximal reabsorption and it effects the removal of NaCl.

First Phase of Proximal Reabsorption. The glomerular ultrafiltrate contains predominantly neutral organic solutes and sodium salts. The filtered neutral organic solute concentration is approximately 10 mM, half of which is glucose and half amino acids. The filtered sodium salt concentration is approximately 140 mM; most of this is NaCl, some is $NaHCO_3$ and a small amount is sodium-coupled to other anions such as acetate, phosphate, citrate, and lactate. All of these solutes are transported from the tubule fluid into the proximal tubule cell by specific carrier complexes which also combine with Na^+ and are thus sodium-coupled secondary active transport processes. To repeat, the Na^+-carrier complex derives the energy to cross the luminal membrane from the electrical and/or chemnical gradient for Na^+. The low intracellular Na^+ concentration is maintained by the Na^+-K^+ ATPase pump

Sodium ion (Na^+) transport in the early proximal tubule.

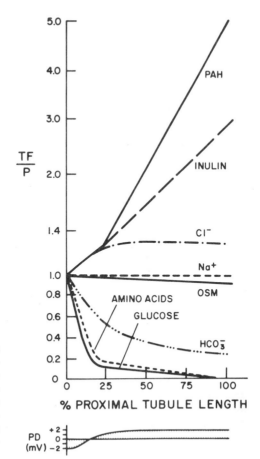

Figure 2–4. Reabsorption of various solutes along the entire proximal tubule in relation to the potential difference (PD). TF/P = tubule fluid-to-plasma concentration ratio. The area above the line for inulin represents solutes that are secreted; the area below the line for inulin represents solutes that are reabsorbed.

system located in the basolateral cell membrane. Representative sodium-coupled transport processes are shown in Figure 2–5 and Table 2–2. These processes are the dominant mechanism by which Na$^+$ enters the proximal tubule cell during the first phase of proximal reabsorption. Once these solutes are transported into the cell their intracellular concentrations are sufficiently great that they may diffuse down their concentration gradient across the basolateral membrane to the peritubular plasma, or they may be metabolized.

The lumen-negative PD in the early proximal tubule is an active transport PD generated by the sodium-coupled reabsorption of glucose and amino acids. These processes generate a PD because they are current-carrying or "electrogenic" and because initially they result in the movement of Na$^+$ from tubule fluid to plasma. Since sodium is a positively charged ion, the blood side of the membrane will become positively charged and the lumen side will become negatively charged. In order to set up this PD only a very few Na$^+$ ions need to move from lumen to blood, just enough to charge the membrane capacitance (about 10^{-12}M). A membrane cannot effect additional separation of charge without movement of the counter ion, in this case Cl$^-$. The proximal tubule is very permeable to Cl$^-$; thus it follows rapidly and the transepithelial PD is low. The other solutes that are reabsorbed in the proximal tubule are electroneutral and do not generate a PD

Differences in potential across the cell membrane can be altered by the movement of a very small number of ions.

Table 2–2. Na⁺ GRADIENT-DEPENDENT TRANSPORT SYSTEMS IN RENAL PROXIMAL TUBULE BRUSH BORDER MEMBRANE VESICLES

Transported Solute	
Sugars	Amino acids *Continued*
D-Glucose	Cystine
D-Galactose	Glycine (L-alanylglycine)
Myoinositol	Ions
Amino acids	Phosphate
Neutral	Sulfate
L-Alanine	Hydroxyl (Na⁺/H⁺ antiport)
L-Phenylalanine	Organic metabolites
L-Glutamine	L-Lactate
Acidic	Ketone bodies
L-Glutamate	Acetoacetate
L-Aspartate	β-Hydroxybutyrate
Basic	Tricarboxylate cycle intermediates
L-Arginine	Succinate
L-Ornithine	α-Ketoglutarate
Imino acids	Citrate
L-Proline	
β-Amino acids	
β-Alanine	
Taurine	

because no net charge crosses the epithelium. For example, lactate reabsorption occurs by sodium-lactate cotransport. Lactate has a negative charge and sodium has a positive charge and since the carrier-complex is neutral, no net charge is transferred.

Water transport follows solute transport in the first phase of proximal reabsorption, driven passively by small osmotic gradients. Recently, small degrees of luminal hypotonicity (3 to 6 mOsm/kg) have been detected in proximal tubule fluid relative to peritubular plasma. The hydraulic water permeability (P_f) of the proximal nephron has been found to range from 0.1 to 0.5 cm/sec. The higher value for P_f (0.5 cm/sec) is consistent with small transepithelial osmotic gradients, on the order of 2 to 5 mOsm, serving as the total driving force for water reabsorption. If on the other hand, the smaller values (e.g., 0.1 cm/sec) represent the true P_f for the proximal tubule, then some osmotic force in addition to luminal hypotonicity must contribute to water reabsorp-

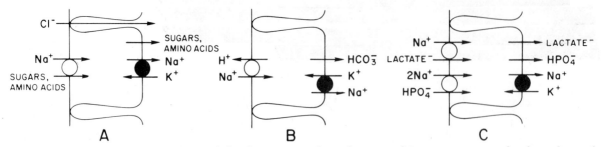

Figure 2–5. Schematic representation of the three principal mechanisms of Na⁺ transport in the first phase of proximal reabsorption. Na⁺ enters the cell by: (A) electrogenic Na⁺ cotransport with neutral organic solutes such as sugars and amino acids; (B) electroneutral Na⁺ countertransport with H⁺; (C) electroneutral Na⁺ cotransport with organic anions. Na⁺ leaves the cell by the Na⁺-K⁺ ATPase pump system. Solutes coupled to Na⁺ transport have elevated intracellular concentrations and leave the cell by passive diffusion.

tion. It has been suggested that Na⁺ transport into the lateral intercellular space raises the salt concentration and thus the osmotic pressure in this local intraepithelial compartment. Since the lateral intercellular spaces are unavailable to experimental observation, it has not been possible to obtain direct information proving or disproving this hypothesis.

Second Phase of Proximal Reabsorption. The second phase of proximal reabsorption effects NaCl reabsorption. In the late proximal tubule there is a high Cl⁻ and a low HCO₃⁻ concentration in the tubule fluid, but there is a normal Cl⁻ and HCO₃⁻ concentration in peritubular plasma. Thus, there are *ion concentration differences*. Since Cl⁻ is the more permeable ion, a lumen-positive transepithelial PD is generated, which serves to retard Cl⁻ and accelerate Na⁺ movement. NaCl reabsorption in the late proximal tubule is both active and passive (Fig. 2–6). The active component accounts for about two thirds of the Na⁺

ACTIVE AND TRANSCELLULAR

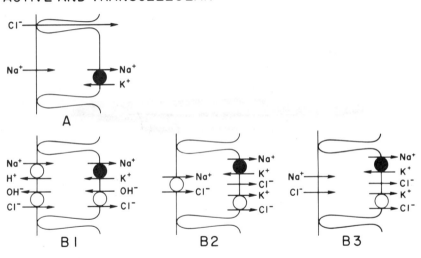

PASSIVE AND PARACELLULAR

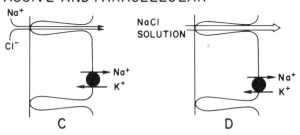

Figure 2–6. Schematic representation of the principal mechanisms of NaCl transport in the second phase of proximal reabsorption. Approximately two thirds of the Na⁺ transport is active and transcellular. It leaves the cell by the Na⁺-K⁺ ATPase pump system. It enters the cell by either "simple" electrogenic Na⁺ transport where Cl⁻ movement is passive and paracellular (A); or electroneutral NaCl transport (B1–B3). Electroneutral Na⁺ and Cl⁻ transport across the luminal membrane might be via parallel Na⁺-H⁺ and Cl⁻-OH⁻ exchangers (B1), NaCl symporter (B2), or parallel Na⁺ and Cl⁻ conductance pathways (B3). One third of the NaCl transport is passive and paracellular. It moves from lumen to blood through the paracellular pathway by either Na⁺ and Cl⁻ diffusion down their electrochemical gradients (C), or the flow of a NaCl solution (convective NaCl movement) (D).

transport and is either uncoupled or traditional active Na^+ transport (panel A, Fig. 2–6) or some form of neutral NaCl transport (panel B, Fig. 2–6). The pathway for Na^+ transport in either case is initially across the luminal cell membrane, driven by the Na^+ concentration gradient, and then across the basolateral cell membrane, driven by the Na^+-K^+ ATPase pump system. The pathway for Cl^- transport either is paracellular, driven by the lumen-negative transepithelial PD for traditional active Na^+ transport, or is transcellular for neutral NaCl transport. At present the mechanism for Cl^- exit from the cell is unknown. It is known that intracellular Cl^- is above electrochemical equilibrium across the basolateral cell membrane, making Cl^- diffusion the simplest possibility. However, the permeability of the basolateral membrane is too low to account for sufficient transport. As an alternative mechanism, a carrier that combines K^+ and Cl^- has been suggested.

There are two possible driving forces for the passive flow of NaCl out of the tubule lumen into the peritubular plasma in the second phase of proximal reabsorption: diffusion and convection (panel C, Fig. 2–6). It should be recalled that these passive forces exist because sugars, amino acids, and HCO_3^- were preferentially reabsorbed by primary and secondary active transport processes in the first phase of proximal reabsorption. Diffusive NaCl reabsorption occurs because there is an electrochemical gradient favoring its movement from lumen to blood. The Cl^- concentration in the tubule fluid is higher than that in blood, which drives Cl^- reabsorption. The transepithelial PD is lumen-positive, which drives Na^+ reabsorption. Convective NaCl reabsorption would occur if the *reflection coefficient** for peritubular plasma solutes such as sugars, amino acids, and $NaHCO_3$ were greater than the reflection coefficient for luminal fluid NaCl. As a result of the difference in reflection coefficients, an effective osmotic pressure difference, capable of driving osmotic water flow, would exist across the proximal tubule epithelium. If the reflection coefficient for NaCl is less than 1.0, some would be drawn along in the water flowing from lumen to blood, thus causing solvent drag or convection of NaCl. This effective osmotic pressure difference might be responsible for some water reabsorption in the second phase of proximal reabsorption.

Capillary Uptake of Proximal Reabsorbate. Once the reabsorbed solute and water are deposited into the lateral intercellular space they rapidly mix with the renal interstitium. Movement from the renal interstitium into the peritubular capillaries is determined by the Starling forces which govern fluid movement across all capillaries (Fig.

NaCl reabsorption in the late proximal tubule.

---

*The term "reflection coefficient" (σ) has been introduced to account for differences in solute permeabilities across biological membranes:

$$\sigma = \Delta\Pi_{obs} / \Delta\Pi_{th}$$

where $\Delta\Pi_{obs}$ is the observed osmotic pressure generated by a solute across a given membrane and $\Delta\Pi_{th}$ is the theoretical osmotic pressure predicted by van't Hoff's law; i.e.,

$$\Delta\Pi = RT\Delta C$$

and ΔC is the solute concentration difference across the membrane. For an ideal nonpermeant solute completely "reflected" by the membrane, $\sigma = 1.0$. For a solute whose permeability approaches that of H_2O, $\sigma = 0$.

Figure 2–7. The peritubular Starling forces influence proximal reabsorption through two mechanisms. First, the net Starling forces across the peritubular capillary (the sum of the colloid osmotic pressure of the capillary minus that of the interstitium (Π_c − Π_I) and the hydraulic pressure of the interstitium minus that of the capillary (P_I − P_c) determine the back-leak of organic solutes through the paracellular pathway (see Fig. 1–13). Second, the interstitial protein concentration in part determines reabsorption of NaCl across the transcellular pathway.

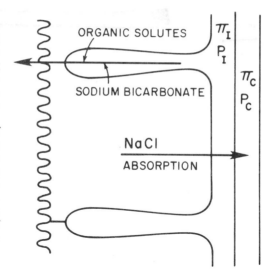

2–7). The reader should refer to the section on Cortical Peritubular Microcirculation in Chapter 1. The Starling forces favoring capillary uptake of reabsorbate are the capillary colloid osmotic pressure and the interstitial hydraulic pressure. The opposing Starling forces are the interstitial colloid osmotic pressure and the capillary hydraulic pressure. The capillary Starling forces are readily altered. Capillary hydraulic pressure is determined by the degree to which the arterial pressure is transmitted through the renal arterioles to the peritubular capillary. Efferent arteriolar dilation allows the peritubular capillary hydraulic pressure to rise; efferent arteriolar constriction increases the pressure drop between glomerular and peritubular capillaries and allows the peritubular hydraulic pressure to fall. Peritubular capillary colloid osmotic pressure is determined by the degree to which the glomerular capillary protein concentration is increased by formation of a glomerular protein-free ultrafiltrate. Thus, the peritubular capillary colloid osmotic pressure is directly related to the glomerular capillary filtration fraction. Usually about 20 percent of the renal plasma flow becomes glomerular ultrafiltrate; thus, the peritubular protein concentration is usually 120 percent of systemic arterial protein concentration. When more of the renal plasma flow is filtered the peritubular protein concentration is proportionally increased.

The Starling forces govern fluid movement across all capillaries.

The uptake of the proximal tubule reabsorbate into the peritubular capillaries is dependent on peritubular Starling forces. When the filtration fraction is increased, peritubular capillary colloid osmotic pressure is increased and peritubular capillary uptake is enhanced. The mechanism for this effect appears to be two-fold. First, the increase in the uptake of reabsorbate is thought to lower the volume of reabsorbate present in the lateral intercellular spaces and decrease the hydraulic pressure in the spaces. Lower lateral intercellular space hydraulic pressure would decrease the width of this compliant compartment. This geometric change would then diminish the permeability of the paracellular transport pathway and reduce back-leak of solutes whose tubule fluid concentrations are lower than that of plasma, such as organic solutes and $NaHCO_3$. A reduction in passive back-leak of reabsorbate into the tubule lumen results in an enhanced net reabsorptive rate. Second, peritubular colloid osmotic pressure appears to directly and proportionately influence neutral transcellular NaCl transport. An increase in peritubular colloid osmotic pressure enhances transcellular NaCl transport. Decreases in peritubular colloid osmotic pressure have the opposite effects; they increase the paracellular permeability and therefore decrease the net reabsorption of solutes whose concentrations fall below plasma, and they specifically inhibit transcellular NaCl reabsorption. The mechanism of the effect of colloid osmotic pressure on transcellular NaCl reabsorption is unknown.

Secretion of Organic Ions. Organic waste products, both cations and anions, are produced by the liver and circulate in the plasma. In addition, numerous exogenous substances and drugs are organic ions; most circulate bound to plasma proteins. Therefore, glomerular ultrafiltration and subsequent absence of tubule reabsorption effectively removes only a small portion of these toxic waste products. The remainder is removed from peritubular plasma by the proximal tubule. The transport of these toxic substances into the tubule fluid is termed *secretion*. Avid tubule secretion lowers the unbound plasma concentration of organic ions and allows the dissociation of organic ions from plasma proteins. Virtually all organic ions and drugs are removed from plasma in one passage through the renal cortex. For a list of secreted organic ions see Table 2–3.

In general, organic ion extraction occurs by an active uphill transport step at the basolateral cell membrane which raises the intracellular organic ion concentration above plasma. The greater permeability of the apical cell membrane allows for passive organic ion diffusion into tubule fluid. The nature of the active step in the basolateral cell membrane is poorly understood, but has been suggested to use the blood-to-cell Na^+ concentration gradient, particularly for organic anions such as para-amino hippurate (PAH). The S2 segment of the proximal tubule is the most important site of organic ion

Essentially all organic ions and drugs are removed from plasma in one passage through the renal cortex.

Table 2–3. ORGANIC MOLECULES SECRETED BY PROXIMAL TUBULES

	Anions	Cations
Endogenous compounds	Bile salts	Acetylcholine
	Cyclic AMP	Choline
	Fatty acids	Creatinine
	Hippurates	Dopamine
	Hydroxybenzoates	Epinephrine
	Hydroxyindoleacetate	Histamine
	Oxalate	Serotonin
	Prostaglandins	Thiamine
	Urate	
Drugs	Acetazolamide	Atropine
	Cephalothin	Cimetidine
	Chlorothiazide	Hexamethonium
	Ethacrynate	Morphine
	Furosemide	Neostigmine
	Penicillin G	Paraquat
	Probenecid	Quinine
	Saccharin	Trimethoprim
	Salicylate	

secretion, probably because it has a greater number of protein carriers in its basolateral cell membrane.

THIN LIMBS OF THE LOOP OF HENLE

The thin limbs of Henle's loop are composed of the thin descending and the thin ascending limbs. Each of these segments has unique passive permeability properties that give it a critical role in urinary concentration and dilution (Fig. 2–8).

The fluid emerging from the proximal nephron is isosmotic to plasma, or about 300 mOsm. The concentration of NaCl in this fluid is about 150 mM and the concentration of urea is about 10 mM. At the end of the proximal nephron, the junction of the outer and inner stripe of the outer zone of the medulla (see Fig. 2–8), the epithelium changes to one with very thin, endothelial-like cells with very few mitochondria. This is the *thin descending limb*. It does not appear to actively transport solutes. The thin descending limb, however, does have unique and interesting passive permeability properties. It is very permeable to water (i.e., has a high osmotic water permeability, L_p), but is relatively impermeable to solutes (low P_s). Thus, when fluid in the thin descending limb is exposed to a hypertonic medullary interstitium, water flows from tubule fluid to interstitium because of the osmotic pressure

The thin descending limb is highly permeable to water but relatively impermeable to urea, Na^+, Cl^- or other solutes.

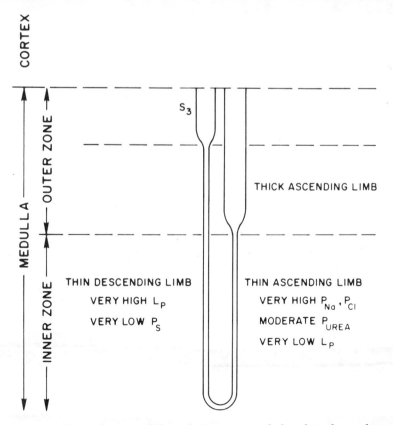

Figure 2–8. Differential permeability characteristics of the thin descending and ascending limbs. L_p, osmotic water permeability; P_s, P_{Na}, P_{Cl}, P_{UREA}, permeability to solutes, Na^+, Cl^- and urea, respectively.

difference and concentrates the tubule fluid NaCl and urea. In water deprivation, enhancement of tubule fluid solute concentration occurs primarily in long-looped nephrons and is about six-fold, from 300 mOsm at the junction of the outer and inner medulla to 1800 mOsm at the tip of the papilla.

The thin ascending limb is water-impermeable, moderately urea-permeable and highly permeable to NaCl.

At the bend of Henle's loop in long-looped nephrons begins the *thin ascending limb*. This tubule segment is similar to the thin descending limb. It also has a thin epithelium without significant mitochondria and as a result is unable to transport solutes actively. In contrast to the thin descending limb, the thin ascending limb is water-impermeable, moderately urea-permeable, and very highly NaCl-permeable. Thus, when fluid in the thin ascending limb is exposed to a hypertonic medullary interstitium the tubule fluid becomes more dilute than the surrounding medullary interstitium. The dilution of the tubule fluid is a result of the permeability characteristics of its membrane and the composition of the tubule fluid emerging from the thin descending limb. During water deprivation the NaCl concentration at the bend of Henle's loop is greater than the surrounding interstitium because of water abstraction in the thin descending limb. The urea concentration in the medullary interstitium is greater than in the tubule fluid because of urea addition from the collecting tubule system. Since the NaCl permeability is greater than the urea permeability, the flow of NaCl out of the thin ascending limb is greater than the flow of urea into the thin ascending limb and the tubule fluid becomes dilute. The absence of any significant water permeability allows the tubule epithelium to maintain the osmotic gradients generated in this fashion.

DISTAL TUBULE SEGMENTS

The main transport function of the distal tubule segments is to transport salt from tubule fluid to interstitium in excess of water. This dilution of the tubule fluid occurs regardless of the state of water balance of the animal and has earned these segments the title of "diluting segments" in some species. In the mammalian nephron the distal tubule segments are divided into two types: the *thick ascending limbs* of Henle's loop and the true *distal convoluted tubule*. These two segments are separated by the area surrounding the macula densa.

The thick ascending limb of Henle's loop begins in the inner stripe of the outer medulla and ends in the area of the macula densa. The epithelium is tall and possesses numerous microvilli and mitochondria. It is generally 3 to 5 mm in length, the longer lengths being achieved in nephrons with more superficial glomeruli. A portion of the thick ascending limb lies in the medulla and a portion lies in the cortex. These two segments function similarly in that they both transport NaCl actively from lumen to interstitium and are impermeable to water and relatively impermeable to urea. The segments have low transepithelial electrical resistances due to high cation permeability of this paracellular pathway. As in the proximal tubule segments, however, the medullary thick limb (the initial segment) transports at a higher rate against lower gradients, whereas the cortical thick limbs transport at lower rates against higher gradients. These differences in transport rate are related to their individual functions. The main function of the medullary segment is to provide for maximal medullary hypertonicity against minimal concentration gradients. A high capacity transport system best effects this result. The main function of the cortical segment is to maximally dilute the tubule fluid. The ability to generate steep concentration gradients best effects this result.

NaCl reabsorption in the thick ascending limb of Henle's loop is a secondary active Na^+ transport process, similar to those occurring in the proximal tubule segments (Fig. 2–9). However, in contrast to the secondary active transport processes in the proximal tubule which generate a lumen-negative or neutral transepithelial potential difference while reabsorbing Na^+, the thick ascending limb generates a lumen-positive potential difference. The mechanism of transcellular NaCl cotransport is shown in Figure 2–9.

There is a transport protein in the luminal membrane that combines two Cl^-, one Na^+, and one K^+ ion. The energy for the translocation of the carrier complex is provided by the chemical concentration gradient for Na^+ and Cl^- between the tubule fluid and the cell cytoplasm. As in the proximal nephron, the low cell Na^+ concentration is maintained by primary active transport via the Na^+-K^+ ATPase pump system located in the basolateral cell membrane. In parallel with the Na^+, K^+, $2Cl^-$ *symporter* in the luminal membrane there is a K^+ diffusion pathway. Thus, at the same time as the symporter moves K^+ across the luminal membrane, K^+ diffuses from the cell back into the tubule fluid. The net effect of this symporter and diffusion pathway is that two Cl^- and one Na^+ move across the luminal cell membrane. The lumen-positive PD is the result of the net excess of negative charge crossing the transcellular pathway. Part of the Na^+ transport

A symporter is a carrier mechanism that transports two or more different ions or molecules simultaneously through a membrane.

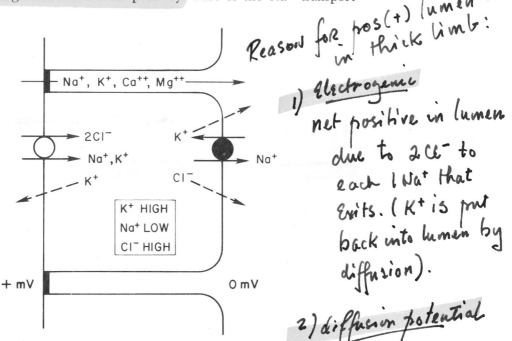

Figure 2–9. Cell model of Na^+, K^+, $2Cl^-$ cotransport in the thick ascending limb of Henle's loop. The lumen-positive PD drives passive cation movement through the cation-selective, low-resistance paracellular pathway.

accompanies the Cl^- across the cellular pathway and part of the Na^+ is driven through the low-resistance paracellular pathway by the lumen-positive PD.

Fluid in the thick ascending limb becomes dilute as salt is reabsorbed from this water-impermeable segment. The lower salt concentration in the tubule fluid relative to the interstitium generates a NaCl dilution potential in addition to the transepithelial PD generated by the secondary active NaCl transport process, the Na^+, K^+, $2Cl^-$ symporter. The thick ascending limb is more permeable to Na^+ than to Cl^- so that the diffusion PD generated is lumen-positive. The sum of the 10 to 20 mV diffusion PD and the 5 to 10 mV transport PD results in a 15 to 30 mV lumen-positive transepithelial PD. An important consequence of the large lumen-positive voltage in the low-resistance thick ascending limb is that large amounts of tubule fluid cations such as K^+, Ca^{++}, and Mg^{++} can be driven from tubule fluid to interstitium passively and thus save cellular metabolic energy.

Numerous diuretics act in the thick ascending limb to inhibit NaCl transport. *Furosemide* is the classic example; it acts rapidly and only from the lumen. It is believed to inhibit active NaCl reabsorption by combining with the symporter in the luminal membrane and preventing its translocation into the cell.

At the junction of the ascending limb and the distal convoluted tubule, the epithelium is somewhat modified and is called the macula densa.

The *macula densa* separates the thick ascending limb from the true distal convoluted tubule. More important, it is the point at which the glomerulus with its afferent and efferent arteriole touches the distal nephron. The macula densa, together with the granular cells of the afferent arteriole, the efferent arterioles, and the extraglomerular mesangium, makes up the *juxtaglomerular apparatus* (see Fig. 1–5). The granular cells of the afferent arteriole are known to secrete renin, the proteolytic enzyme essential for the production of angiotensin II. Macula densa cells are specialized to function as a sensor of transport events up to the distal convoluted tubule and as a messenger of these transport events to the granular cells of the afferent arteriole. It is believed that the macula densa cells transport NaCl from tubule fluid into their cytoplasm in order to equalize the concentrations in both the cell and the tubule fluid. The tubule macula densa cells and the granular cells in the smooth muscle of the afferent arteriole are not separated by an intact basement membrane and the macula densa cells send cytoplasmic projections into the granular cells. The *Golgi apparatus* is located within these projections. Thus, it is believed that these two cell types are acting as a syncytium. When the NaCl concentration in the tubule fluid is low, systemic renin release is activated, ultimately leading to stimulation of aldosterone and Na^+ conservation.

The distal convoluted tubule possesses the highest Na^+-K^+ ATPase activity of any nephron segment.

The osmolality of the tubule fluid emerging from the thick ascending limb is about half that of plasma, or 150 mOsm. The distal convoluted tubule, which begins 0.1 to 0.2 mm beyond the macula densa and extends 0.8 mm at most, continues the active dilution of the tubule fluid begun by the thick ascending limb, but it uses a more traditional Na^+ transport mechanism. The distal convoluted tubule generates a ouabain-sensitive, lumen-negative, transepithelial PD and possesses the highest activity of Na^+-K^+ ATPase of any of the nephron segments. Both of these factors indicate that this tubule segment is importantly involved in transcellular Na^+ transport. In addition, it is very impermeable to water. Thus, NaCl reabsorption proceeds in the absence of water movement and the tubule fluid is further diluted. Interestingly, the distal convoluted tubule is also the major site of action of the hormone calcitonin, which is believed to stimulate adenylate cyclase and somehow to enhance Ca^{++} reabsorption in this segment.

COLLECTING TUBULE SEGMENTS

The collecting tubule segments begin in the outer cortex before the confluence of two adjacent tubules and extend into the calyx of the renal pelvis. Two extremely short segments are present before the confluence, the connecting tubule and the initial cortical collecting tubule. After the confluence the collecting tubule descends, increasing in diameter because of the confluence with other nephrons.

The connecting tubule is an intermediate segment similar to the distal convoluted tubule in that it has a lumen-negative transepithelial PD, a high Na^+-K^+ ATPase activity and a very low water permeability. It differs from the distal convoluted tubule in that it shows sensitivity to several hormones. The physiological response to parathyroid hormone is believed to be involved in the Ca^{++} transport known to occur in this segment; the physiological response to other hormones is unknown.

The collecting tubule segments are the important sites for the final regulation of urinary Na^+, K^+, H^+, water, and urea excretion (Table 2–4). These various transport functions are probably not performed by each cell in the collecting tubule.

The collecting tubule segments contain two cell types: the *principal* or light cells and the *intercalated* or dark cells (Fig. 2–10). The morphology of the intercalated cells is clearly different from the principal. The intercalated cells feature a dark cytoplasm, numerous large mitochondria and other cell organelles, and a striking assortment of prominent ridges on the apical surface. The principal cells, on the other hand, have a light cytoplasm, fewer intracellular organelles, and a single long cilium projecting into the lumen from an apical membrane with short, blunt microvilli (Fig. 2–10). There is, however, a change in both of these cell types as they descend toward the papilla. The number of intercalated cells decreases gradually, so that there are few, if any, in the papillary or inner medullary zone of the kidney. The principal cells increase from cortex to papilla and, more important,

Table 2–4. TRANSPORT FUNCTIONS OF
COLLECTING TUBULE SEGMENTS

	Na^+ Absorption	Cl^- Absorption	K^+ Absorption	K^+ Secretion	H^+ Secretion	HCO_3^- Secretion
Cortical collecting tubule	+ + +	+ +	+ + +	+ + +	+ +	+ +
Medullary collecting tubule	+ /0	+ /0	+ /0	+ /0	+ + + +	?
Papillary collecting tubule	+ + +	+ +	?	?	+	?

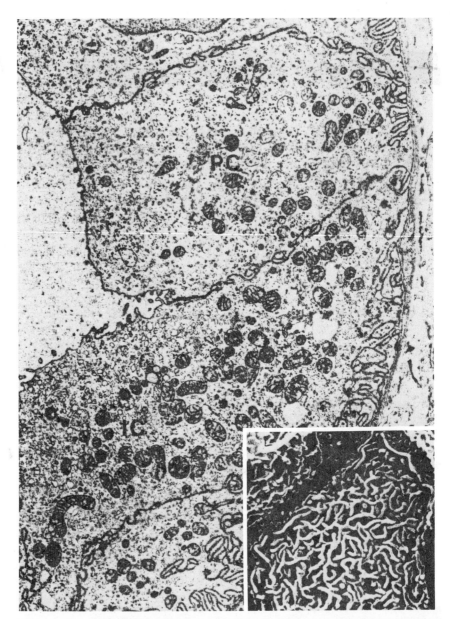

Figure 2–10. Transmission electron micrograph of a human cortical collecting duct. Note the intercalated (IC) or dark cells with their many mitochondria, and the principal (PC) or light cells with their few mitochondria (× 7,000). The inset shows a scanning electron micrograph of the surface of an intercalated cell from the rabbit kidney (× 8,000). (From Bulger, R. E., and Dobyan, D. C.: Recent advances in renal morphology. Ann. Rev. Physiol. 44:147–180, 1982, with permission.)

there appears to be a dramatic change in the *carbonic anhydrase* content of the cells (Table 2–5).

Since it is not possible to subdivide the collecting tubule segments on the basis of cell type it is common to distinguish between portions of the collecting tubule on the basis of their location in the kidney: cortical, medullary, and papillary collecting tubule.

**Table 2–5. DISTRIBUTION OF COLLECTING SEGMENT
CELL TYPES AND CARBONIC ANHYDRASE (CA)**

	Principal Cells		Intercalated Cells	
	Percent Total Cells	*CA*	*Percent Total Cells*	*CA*
Cortical collecting tubule	70–80	0	20–30	+
Medullary collecting tubule	>90	+	<10	+
Papillary collecting tubule	100	+/0	0	0

NaCl Transport. In the collecting tubule the active transport mechanism reabsorbs Na^+ to extremely low levels (Fig. 2–11, panel A). During states of Na^+ deprivation the urinary Na^+ concentration can be as low as 1 mEq. The Na^+ permeability in the luminal membrane allows sodium to enter the cell down its concentration gradient where it is maintained by the Na^+-K^+ ATPase pump system. Low tubule fluid Na^+ concentrations are achievable because the paracellular pathway in the collecting tubule system is very poorly permeable. It is said to have a high electrical resistance. Because of the high paracellular resistance in the collecting tubule segments, Cl^- follows with difficulty and the reabsorption of Na^+ generates a large lumen-negative electrical

The reabsorption of Na^+ takes place by active mechanism, while water and Cl^- are passively reabsorbed.

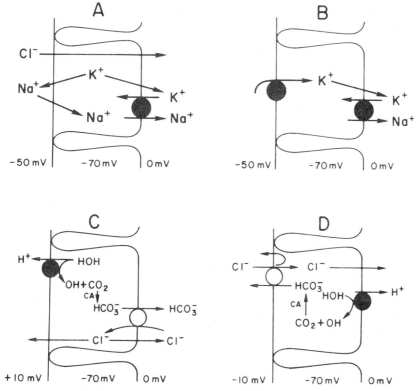

Figure 2–11. Collecting duct transport functions. (A) Na^+ and Cl^- reabsorption and K^+ secretion; (B) K^+ reabsorption; (C) H^+ secretion; (D) HCO_3^- secretion. Closed circles represent pumps requiring metabolic energy. Open circles represent passive ion carriers.

potential difference. The cortical and papillary collecting tubules predominantly reabsorb NaCl. The rate of Na^+ reabsorption in the tubules is approximately the same as the later portion of the proximal nephron, and is controlled by *mineralocorticoid hormones* such as aldosterone. Both the cortical and papillary segments feature principal cells without carbonic anhydrase, suggesting that this cell type might be responsible for NaCl reabsorption.

K^+ Transport. Most (90 to 95 percent) of filtered K^+ is reabsorbed before the tubule fluid reaches the collecting tubules, which are thus the source of K^+ in the urine. The collecting tubule is capable of both K^+ reabsorption and active K^+ secretion, depending on dietary intake. Both the principal and the intercalated cells show specific morphologic alteration when potassium intake is changed, suggesting that the transport functions of K^+ secretion and reabsorption are spatially separated. The principal cells appear morphologically to increase their basolateral infoldings when K^+ secretion is stimulated by chronic K^+ loading and therefore are believed to be responsible for K^+ secretion. The intercalated cells appear morphologically to increase the density of rod-shaped particles in their luminal membranes when K^+ reabsorption is stimulated by dietary potassium restriction. The dark cells are, therefore, believed to be responsible for K^+ reabsorption. This separation of K^+ reabsorption and secretion into different cell types is practical because reabsorption and secretion require markedly different membrane characteristics.

The light (or principal) cell in the collecting tubule is responsible for K^+ secretion and Na^+ reabsorption.

The collecting tubule cell responsible for K^+ secretion, the light or principal cell, is the same as that responsible for Na^+ reabsorption and is shown in Figure 2–11, panel A. The active step in K^+ secretion is the Na^+-K^+ ATPase pump system located in the basolateral cell membrane. This active transport system creates a high intracellular K^+ concentration in these cells. The cells responsible for K^+ secretion are, however, different from other cells in one important respect. The passive K^+ permeability of the apical membrane is much greater than the passive permeability of the basolateral cell membrane. Thus, although the high intracellular K^+ concentration favors diffusion of K^+ from cell into lumen and back into interstitial fluid, the greater K^+ permeability of the luminal membrane ensures that most K^+ diffuses from cell to lumen and that K^+ secretion occurs. The collecting tubule cells responsible for K^+ reabsorption, the intercalated or dark cells, are depicted in Figure 2–11, panel B. There is a primary active K^+ transport system located in the luminal cell membrane, and, in contrast to the principal cells, the K^+ permeability of the luminal cell membrane is very low. As a result, the high intracellular K^+ concentration generates K^+ diffusion across the basolateral membrane and K^+ reabsorption.

With K^+ reabsorption and secretion present in the same tubule segment, it is sometimes difficult to define which process is being affected. For example, net K^+ secretion might be reduced by enhancing K^+ reabsorption or reducing K^+ secretion. For the most part, K^+ reabsorption has been assumed to be constant and alterations in K^+ excretion are believed to be due entirely to changes in K^+ secretion. Some recent evidence, however, may be challenging this point.

H^+ and HCO_3^- Transport. All segments of the collecting tubule are able to acidify the tubule fluid, although the medullary collecting tubule acidifies best. Since the permeability of the paracellular pathway decreases from cortex to papilla, the ability of the collecting tubule segments to establish an H^+ concentration gradient increases from cortex to papilla. The pH in the cortical segment reaches about 6.0 and is sufficient to titrate the bulk of the filtered phosphate buffer. The pH in the medullary collecting tubule reaches about 5.0 and is most important for trapping of medullary ammonia for excretion. The pH in the papillary segments can go below 5.0, to perhaps 4.0. This is clearly the largest ion concentration gradient generated in the kidney. To view this more easily, consider that the pH of plasma is 7.4 and is equivalent to an H^+ concentration of 40 nmol/liter. For a tubule fluid pH of 4.4, the H^+ concentration is 40 μmol/liter. The ratio of H^+ concentration for these fluids is 1:1000.

The mechanism of H^+ secretion in the collecting tubule segments is a primary active transport system located on the luminal cell membrane of the intercalated cells. The cell model responsible for tubule fluid acidification is shown in Figure 2–11, panel C. The H^+ pump is believed to be a proton-translocating ATPase, which splits ATP and releases H^+ into the tubule fluid and OH^- into the cell cytoplasm. Acidification requires carbonic anhydrase in order to accelerate the intracellular buffering of the OH^- with CO_2. The transfer of positive charge into the lumen results in the generation of a lumen-positive transepithelial potential difference. Tubule fluid acidification can also be secondarily affected by the lumen-negative PD generated by Na^+ transport. A large lumen-negative PD would enhance H^+ transport through the pump. The HCO_3^- exits the cell via an electroneutral Cl^--HCO_3^- exchanger in the basolateral cell membrane. The Cl^- can either move across the apical membrane or recycle back across the basolateral cell membrane.

The dark (or intercalated) cells contain a proton-translocating ATPase on their luminal membranes and therefore are capable of secreting H^+ ions. A subpopulation of these cells exhibit reversed polarity and secrete HCO_3^-.

A subpopulation of the intercalated cells of the cortical collecting tubule segments can also secrete HCO_3^-, depending on the acid-base status of the animal. Ability to excrete an alkaline urine is important when dietary intake is alkaline, as is the case for most vegetarians. A subpopulation of the intercalated cells of the collecting tubule have been shown to secrete HCO_3^-. These cells are probably reversed in polarity from those that secrete protons and function as shown in Figure 2–11, panel D.

Water Transport. The collecting tubule segments all participate in the formation of a concentrated urine and in the maintenance of a dilute urine. In the absence of *antidiuretic hormone (ADH)*, they are all poorly permeable to water, although the papillary collecting duct retains some residual water permeability. Continued Na^+ transport along these segments without water reabsorption results in a urinary osmolality of about 50 mOsm. In the presence of ADH, all the collecting tubule segments become highly permeable to water. The maximal urine osmolality is about 1300 mOsm.

In the collecting tubule segments, ADH controls water transport by altering the hydraulic permeability of the collecting tubule cells.

Urea Transport. Urea transport in the collecting tubule segments is entirely passive. The unique permeability characteristics, however, are very important for the efficient operation of the countercurrent system. The urea permeability of the collecting tubule segments is unaltered by antidiuretic hormone, both the cortical and the medullary collecting tubules are essentially impermeable to urea, and the papillary collecting ducts are permeable to urea. The low permeability of the cortical and medullary collecting tubule prevents the loss of recycled urea in the cortex and ensures its delivery to the papilla. The high urea permeability of the papillary collecting tubule enables the recycled urea to enter the medullary interstitium where it facilitates the concentrating function of the thin limbs of Henle's loop.

Mineralocorticoid Hormone Control of Na⁺, K⁺, and H⁺ Transport. The transport of the principal salts in the collecting tubule segments is controlled by mineralocorticoids, such as *aldosterone*. Aldosterone is produced by the zona glomerulosa of the adrenal cortex. It stimulates Na^+ reabsorption, K^+ secretion, and H^+ secretion. Although mineralocorticoids have direct control over only a small proportion of the filtered salts, their influence is critical to maintenance of salt balance. For example, the total quantity of Na^+ reabsorbed under the influence of aldosterone is approximately 2 percent of the filtered load; in the complete absence of aldosterone, one would excrete 2 percent of the filtered Na^+. In the presence of maximal plasma concentrations of aldosterone, virtually no Na^+ is excreted. Two percent of the filtered load amounts to about 33.4 gm/day, roughly three times the normal dietary intake.

Aldosterone acts on the collecting tubule segments to increase K^+ and H^+ secretion and Na^+ reabsorption. Its effect on K^+ secretion is at least in part immediate, while the effect on H^+ and Na^+ requires a 60- and 90-minute latent period, respectively. As shown in Figure 2–12, aldosterone enters the cells of the collecting tubule by diffusion across the basolateral cell membrane and combines in the cell cytoplasm with a receptor to form an *active steroid receptor complex*, which then enters the cell nucleus. The active complex induces the transcription of both messenger and ribosomal RNA, which leads to increased production of an *aldosterone-induced protein*. The induced protein mediates some of the physiological effects of the steroid.

The induced protein has two primary physiological effects (Table 2–6). First, it directly stimulates primary active H^+ secretion. Second, it stimulates cell metabolism. The stimulation of cell metabolism appears to increase Na^+ permeability of the luminal cell membrane, which results in an increased cell Na^+ concentration. The increased cell Na^+ concentration stimulates the activity of the Na^+-K^+ ATPase pump system, which in turn stimulates Na^+ reabsorption and increases intracellular K^+ concentration. Enhanced cell K^+ amplifies the already increased K^+ secretion induced by the immediate effect of the steroid on K^+ permeability.

Antidiuretic Hormone Control of Water Transport. The water permeability of the apical cell membrane of the collecting tubule cells is controlled by *vasopressin* or ADH. ADH is an octapeptide produced by a discrete group of hypothalamic neurons whose cell bodies are located in the supraoptic and paraventricular nuclei and whose axons terminate in the posterior pituitary, from which ADH is released into the blood. In the presence of ADH the entire collecting tubule system becomes permeable to water and the kidney is able to take advantage

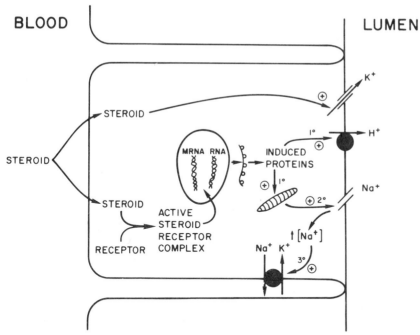

BLOOD   LUMEN

Figure 2–12. Model for the mechanism of action of aldosterone. The steroid hormone enters the collecting tubule cell by diffusion. Hormone directly increases the K^+ permeability of the luminal membrane thereby enhancing K^+ secretion. It also combines with a cytoplasmic receptor. The active steroid receptor complex is translocated to the nucleus where it interacts to stimulate messenger RNA (mRNA) and ribosomal RNA (rRNA) transcription. mRNA and rRNA direct the increased translation of the hormone-induced protein. The induced protein directly ($1°$) increases the activity of the H^+ pump and the supply of energy from the mitochondria. The increased energy supply appears to increase the Na^+ permeability of the luminal membrane which in turn increases cell Na^+ concentration and stimulates the Na^+-K^+ ATPase pump system.

of the osmotic pressure gradient between the concentrated medullary interstitium and the dilute collecting tubule fluid. Urine osmolality in humans can reach 1300 mOsm and urine volume can be as little as 0.5 liter/day.

ADH increases the water permeability of the collecting tubule segments by attaching to a specific receptor on the basolateral membrane of the principal cells of the collecting tubule (Fig. 2–13). This hormone-receptor complex activates *adenyl cyclase*, resulting in the generation of *cyclic AMP* from ATP. In the collecting tubule cells cyclic

Table 2–6. EFFECTS OF MINERALOCORTICOID HORMONE IN COLLECTING TUBULE SEGMENTS

Immediate	Latent via Induced Protein		
↑ luminal membrane potassium permeability	$1°$	↑	proton pump activity
	$1°$	↑	metabolism
	$2°$	↑	luminal membrane Na^+ permeability
	$3°$	↑	Na^+–K^+ ATPase pump activity

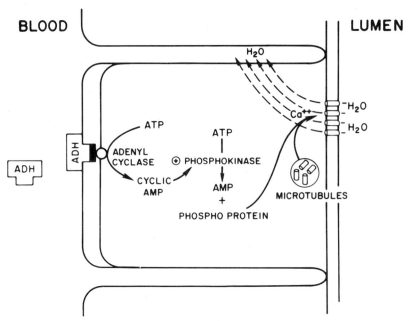

Figure 2–13. Model for the cellular action of ADH. ADH binds to a receptor on the peritubular surface of the collecting tubule cell where, in the presence of ATP, adenyl cyclase generates cyclic AMP. Cyclic AMP stimulates a phosphokinase that phosphorylates a protein which, in the presence of Ca^{++}, inserts preformed "water channels" into the apical cell membrane.

AMP activates a phosphokinase which, in the presence of Ca^{++} and ATP, phosphorylates a protein that increases the water permeability of the apical cell membrane. It is likely that the phosphorylated protein is in some way involved with intracellular microtubules and microfilaments within "channel-containing cytosolic vacuoles." Insertions of these channel-containing membrane patches show up as intramembranous particles or aggregates in freeze-fracture electron microscopy. The inserted water channels behave as if they had a radius of about 2 Å because they allow water, but not solutes, to penetrate.

URINE CONCENTRATION AND DILUTION

In order to maintain water balance, the volume and osmolality of the urine must be controlled. Control is achieved by ADH. In times of excess water intake, the kidney excretes a dilute urine and thus rids the body of its excess water. In humans the greatest rate of urine flow is about 1.5 liters/hr, approximately 20 percent of the glomerular filtration rate, with an osmolality of 50 mOsm. This means that of the 180 liters of plasma filtered per day only about 36 are under ADH control. The remaining 144 liters are obligatorily coupled to solute reabsorption. *Obligatory water reabsorption* occurs primarily in the proximal tubule and the thin descending limb of Henle's loop. Some water reabsorption also occurs in the distal tubule and collecting tubule segments because they are not completely impermeable to water. The lowest osmolality achievable is finite because of obligatory solute excretion, because of the failure of salt reabsorptive processes, and because of the finite tubule water permeability. In times of water deprivation, the kidney excretes a maximally concentrated urine and thus returns filtered water to the body fluids. In the human kidney the maximum achieveable osmolality is about 1300 mOsm. There is an obligatory waste product excretion of substances like urea, sulfate, and phosphate amounting to about 600 mOsm/day. This means that at least 0.5 liter of water per day must be excreted by the kidney.

It is relatively easy to visualize the elaboration of a dilute urine. In the absence of ADH the water permeability of the collecting tubule segments is small, but salt reabsorption continues in the thick ascending limb of Henle's loop, the distal tubule, and the collecting tubule segments. Salt reabsorption in the absence of water reabsorption progressively dilutes the tubule fluid below plasma levels. The urine is dilute.

Formation of dilute urine is a relatively simple process, but concentration of urine takes place by the complex "countercurrent" mechanism.

It is more difficult to imagine how the kidney forms a concentrated urine. The urine could be concentrated by active water transport from tubule fluid to blood in the collecting tubule system, which would require a tremendous expenditure of metabolic energy. In fact it requires more than 300 times the energy needed by active salt transport and passive water equilibration because salt concentrations are on the order of 0.15 M, while water concentrations are about 55 M. Instead, urine is concentrated with relatively little expenditure of metabolic energy by a complex interaction between the loops of Henle, the medullary interstitium, the medullary blood vessels or vasa recta, and the collecting tubule. This mechanism of urine concentration is called the *countercurrent mechanism* because of the anatomic arrangement of these tubule and vascular elements. Tubule fluid moves from the cortex down into the medulla toward the papillary tip via the proximal straight tubule and the thin descending limbs. The tubules then loop back toward the cortex so that the direction of fluid movement is reversed in the ascending limbs. Similarly, the vasa recta descends to the tip of the papilla and then loops back toward the cortex. The arrangement of tubule segments and vasa recta allows for the two fundamental processes of the countercurrent mechanism to take place: *countercurrent multiplication* and *countercurrent exchange.*

Countercurrent multiplication occurs in the loop of Henle and requires specific permeability and transport characteristics of the descending and ascending limbs (Table 2–7). The ascending limb must

Table 2–7. PERMEABILITY AND TRANSPORT PROPERTIES OF TUBULE SEGMENTS INVOLVED IN URINE CONCENTRATION (ADH MAXIMAL)

	Active Salt Transport	Permeability		
		H_2O	*Urea*	*NaCl*
Thin DLH	0	+ + + +	+	±
Thin ALH	0	±	+	+ + +
Thick ALH	+ + + +	±	±	±
Distal convoluted tubule	+	±	0	±
Cortical collecting tubule	+	+ + +	0	±
Outer medullary collecting tubule	+	+ + +	0	±
Papillary collecting tubule	+	+ + +	+ + +	±

DLH, descending limb of Henle; ALH, ascending limb of Henle.

possess an active transport process capable of generating a concentration gradient and it must be *water-impermeable*. The active transport process thus dilutes the tubule fluid in the ascending limb and concentrates the medullary interstitium. The descending limb needs only to be *water-permeable* so that its tubule fluid can equilibrate with the hypertonic medullary interstitium. The principle of countercurrent multiplication is shown in Figure 2–14, where ascending and descending limbs are separated by the interstitium and transport and flow are considered separate processes. Initially all fluids have an osmolality of 300 mOsm. In the figure's second panel active transport in the ascending limb generates a 200 mOsm gradient between ascending limb fluid and interstitium; the descending limb fluid equilibrates with the interstitium. In panels three through six these processes are repeated. In panel six the fluid in the ascending limb is 400 mOsm at the tip and 125 mOsm at the base. The base-to-tip osmotic concentration gradient is 275 mOsm, which is greater than the 200 mOsm

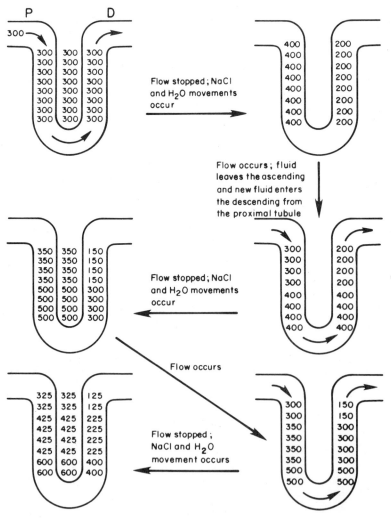

Figure 2–14. Countercurrent multiplication system in the loop of Henle. (Redrawn from Pitts, R. F.: Physiology of the Kidney and Body Fluids, 3rd Edition. Year Book Medical Publishers, Chicago, 1974.)

maximal gradient generated at any level in the loop structure. This enhancement of the maximal gradient generated by countercurrent flow is countercurrent multiplication. It is possible to enhance the multiplication manyfold by increasing the number of transport and flow sequences and by increasing the length of the loops used.

This form of countercurrent multiplication, which is dependent on active transport of salt, occurs primarily in the thick ascending limbs located in the outer medulla. In contrast, the thin limbs of Henle's loop, which are located in the inner medulla, are incapable of active salt transport. In the inner medulla and papilla, therefore, countercurrent multiplication occurs by passive processes, using urea recycling (Fig. 2–15). In this region of the kidney urea constitutes at least half of the medullary interstitial solute. The thin descending limb is highly permeable to water and poorly permeable to urea and salt. As the isotonic salt solution leaves the proximal tubule and passes through the

Countercurrent multiplication occurs in the loop of Henle, while countercurrent exchange takes place in the vasa recta. Together they make up the mechanism by which urine is concentrated.

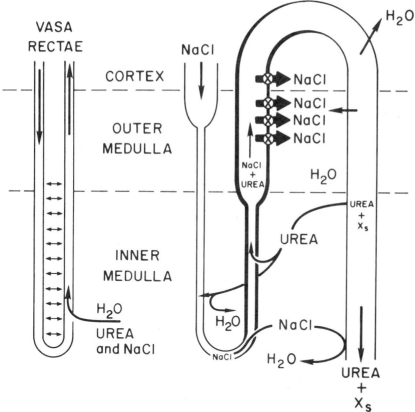

Figure 2–15. Schematics of countercurrent multiplication and exchange system without active transport in the renal inner medulla. Countercurrent multiplication occurs in the loops of Henle. Fluid entering the descending limb is isosmotic. The ascending limb is water-impermeable (denoted by heavy black line) and possesses an active NaCl transport process, thus diluting the tubule fluid and concentrating the medullary interstitium. The solute gradient is multiplied from base to tip because of countercurrent flow. The descending limb and collecting tubule are water-permeable; thus their tubule fluid equilibrates osmotically with the hypertonic medullary interstitium. Urea recycling greatly enhances medullary hypertonicity, and medullary urea provides for NaCl concentration gradients across the ascending thin limb and passive dilution in this segment. Countercurrent exchange in the vasa recta prevents dissipation of medullary hypertonicity by blood flow wash-out. X_s is nonreabsorbable solutes.

thin descending limb, osmotic equilibration occurs by water abstraction. As a consequence, the NaCl concentration in the loop fluid rises above the NaCl concentration in the medullary interstitium. The fluid then enters the thin ascending limb, which is water-impermeable, modestly permeable to urea, and highly permeable to NaCl. As a consequence, NaCl diffuses out of the thin ascending limb down its concentration gradient faster than urea diffuses into the lumen down its concentration gradient. Further, solute in the form of salt is added to the inner medullary interstitium and the luminal fluid is diluted. The urea that enters the thin ascending limb remains in the tubule fluid as it transits the thick ascending limb, distal convoluted tubule, connecting tubule, cortical collecting tubule, and outer medullary collecting tubule, and is recycled to the medullary interstitium via diffusion out of the inner medullary and papillary collecting tubules.

Countercurrent exchange occurs in the vasa recta and is equally important to the operation of the countercurrent mechanism (Fig. 2–16). The reader is referred to the section on the Medullary Microcirculation in Chapter 1. Water and solutes are freely permeable across capillaries. Thus, as blood descends into an area of higher osmolality, solutes can move into and water can move out of the vessels. If the vasa recta entered from the cortex, descended into the medulla, and then exited from the kidney, they would carry out medullary interstitial solutes. Because they ascend back toward the cortex into a region of progressively lower osmolality, solutes move back out of the vessels and water moves back into them. Vasa recta thus exhibit countercurrent exchange which preserves medullary interstitial osmolality.

The entire purpose of countercurrent multiplication in the loops of Henle and exchange in the vasa recta is to create a hypertonic medullary interstitium. In the presence of a hypertonic interstitium and ADH, the collecting tubule segments can concentrate the urine by passive water equilibration. Urea augments medullary interstitial

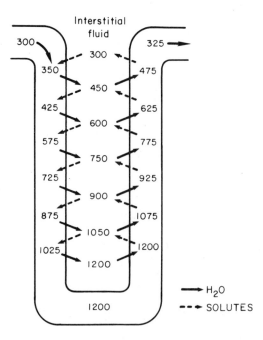

Figure 2–16. Vasa recta as countercurrent exchangers. (Redrawn from Pitts, R. F.: Physiology of the Kidney and Body Fluids, 3rd Edition. Year Book Medical Publishers, Chicago, 1974.)

osmolality. Filtered urea is raised to high levels by the bend of the loop of Henle because of obligatory water abstraction in both the proximal tubule segments and the descending limb of Henle's loop. In the presence of ADH water abstraction continues to increase the tubule fluid urea concentration if the collecting tubule segments are impermeable to urea, but the papillary collecting tubule is urea-permeable. The high urea concentration in the tubule fluid is dissipated and urea is added to the medullary interstitium. About 50 percent of the medullary interstitial osmolality is made up of urea. Most of the medullary interstitial urea enters the ascending thin limb of Henle's loop and is recycled back to the collecting tubules. Urea recycling preserves medullary interstitial urea, thus aiding in maintaining medullary interstitial hypertonicity and urine concentration.

REFERENCES

Anatomy

Bulger, R. E., and Dobyan, D. C.: Recent advances in renal morphology. Ann. Rev. Physiol. 44:147–180, 1982.
Overview of the most recent scanning and transmission electron micrographs of the renal nephron.

Kaissling, B., and Kriz, W.: Structural analysis of the rabbit kidney. *In* Advances in Anatomy, Embryology and Cell Biology. Springer-Verlag, New York, 1978.
"The" complete anatomical guide to the rabbit nephron. Perhaps too complete for all but the serious investigator.

Basic Mechanism of Transport

Hebert, S. C., Schafer, J. A., and Andreoli, T. E.: Principles of membrane transport. *In* Brenner, B. M., and Rector, F. C., Jr., eds.: The Kidney, 2nd Edition. W. B. Saunders Co., Philadelphia, 1981.
Basic membrane transport written for the physician and graduate student in biology.

Aronson, P. S.: Identifying secondary active transport in epithelia. Am. J. Physiol. 45:F1–F11, 1981.
Good definitions of primary versus secondary active transport. Better identification of all secondary processes.

Proximal Tubule

Rector, F. C., Jr.: Sodium, bicarbonate, and chloride absorption by the proximal tubule. Am. J. Physiol. 244:F461–F471, 1983.
Review of recent work on proximal $NaHCO_3$ and NaCl transport and their physiologic control. In general somewhat advanced.

Berry, C. A., and Warnock, D. G.: Acidification in the in vitro perfused tubule. Kidney Int. 22:507–518, 1982.
Basic review of acidification in proximal and distal nephron segments. Easy description of data, but somewhat outdated.

Berry, C. A.: Water permeability and pathways in the proximal tubule. Am. J. Physiol. 245:F279–F294, 1983.
Basic theoretical and critical review of the mechanism of water transport in the proximal tubule.

Berry, C. A., and Rector, F. C., Jr.: Active and passive sodium transport in the proximal tubule. Miner. Electrolyte Metab. 4:149–160, 1980.
Basic review of the mechanism of proximal sodium transport. Readable for the most part. Old but not that outdated.

Berry, C. A.: Lack of effect of peritubular protein on passive NaCl transport in the rabbit proximal tubule. J. Clin. Invest. 71:268–281, 1983.
Original study examining the control of proximal transport by peritubular physical factors.

Grantham, J. J.: Studies of organic anion and cation transport in isolated segments of proximal tubules. Kidney Int. 22:519–525, 1982.
Review of original work by the author and others on the important proximal secretory processes.

Thin Limbs of the Loop of Henle

Kokko, J. P.: Transport characteristics of the thin limbs of Henle. Kidney Int. 22:449–453, 1982.
A clear review of original work by the author. Important for understanding the mechanism of urinary concentration and dilution.

Distal Tubule Segments

Burg, M. B.: Thick ascending limb of Henle's loop. Kidney Int. 22:454–464, 1982.
Review of original work by the author and others. Clear, but becoming outdated. Combine with Greger et al. below.

Burg, M. B., and Good, D.: Sodium chloride coupled transport in mammalian nephrons. Ann. Rev. Physiol. 45:533–547, 1983.
Review of NaCl coupled processes throughout the nephron with emphasis on the thick ascending limb.

Greger, R., Schlatter, E., and Lang, F.: Evidence for electroneutral sodium chloride cotransport in the cortical thick ascending limb of Henle's loop of rabbit kidney. Pflugers Arch. 396:308–314, 1983.
Original study.

Imai, M., and Nakamura, R.: Function of distal convoluted and connecting tubules studied by isolated nephron fragments. Kidney Int. 22:465–472, 1982.
Review of original work by the only group that can look at distal convoluted and connecting tubule function.

Collecting Tubule Segments

Stokes, J. B.: Ion transport by the cortical and outer medullary collecting tubule. Kidney Int. 22:473–484, 1982.
Review of the author's original work. Good for Na and K, not so good for H.

Stone, D. K., Seldin, D. W., Kokko, J. P., and Jacobson, H. R.: Anion dependence of rabbit medullary collecting duct acidification. J. Clin. Invest. 71:1505–1508, 1983.
Original study.

Urine Concentration and Dilution

Kokko, J. P., and Rector, F. C., Jr.: Countercurrent multiplication system without active transport in inner medulla. Kidney Int. 2:214–223, 1972.
Classic presentation of passive countercurrent system.

Jamison, R. L., and Kriz, W.: Urinary Concentrating Mechanism: Structure and Function. Oxford University Press, New York, 1982.
More than you ever wanted to know about urinary concentration.

Handler, J. S., and Orloff, J.: Antidiuretic hormone. Ann. Rev. Physiol. 43:611–624, 1981.
Dated but short review of original work. Not especially clear, but a good reference source.

Regulation of Body Fluid Tonicity

Regulation of body fluid tonicity depends largely on the regulation of body water content. Water deficits give rise to increased concentration of solutes and *hypertonicity* of body fluids, while water surfeits result in a *hypotonic* state. Normally the tonicity of the body fluids is maintained within very narrow limits by the complementary action of several physiologic control mechanisms including thirst, antidiuretic hormone (ADH) secretion, and ADH action on the kidney to promote renal water conservation. This fine degree of regulation presumably reflects an important dependence of many cellular processes on optimal cell volumes and solute concentrations. When these normal control mechanisms become disordered, a variety of organ systems, particularly the central nervous system, may suffer abnormalities of function and thus compound the initial disorder. In order to identify and appropriately treat these disturbances of tonicity, an appreciation of the normal control mechanisms is critical.

ANATOMY OF THE BODY FLUIDS

Total body water content amounts to about 50 percent of body weight in adult females and 60 percent of body weight in adult males. This volume of fluid is divided into two major compartments: *extracellular* and *intracellular* (Fig. 3–1). The latter is the larger and contains about two thirds of the total body water, with the extracellular compartment accounting for the other one third. Extracellular fluid is further compartmentalized into an *interstitial* space that contains about three fourths of the extracellular fluid volume, while the *plasma volume* comprises the remaining one quarter. Finally, a very small portion of the total body fluid is considered *transcellular* and consists of the various secretions within the gastrointestinal tract, fluids present in synovial spaces, and cerebrospinal and ocular fluids.

Fluid Movement Between Intracellular and Extracellular Compartments. The normal composition of the various body fluid spaces is depicted in Figure 3–2. As can be seen, the extracellular solutes consist principally of Na^+, with Cl^- and HCO_3^- as the attendant anions, while the intracellular solutes include K^+ and Mg^{++}, with phosphates and proteins as the dominant anions. The mechanism by which solute composition is regulated is the cell membrane's ability to either exclude specific solutes (on the basis of size or charge) or pump specific solutes into or out of the cell interior, as discussed in detail in Chapter 2.

While water moves freely across virtually all cell membranes, tonicity of the extracellular fluid is determined by its concentration of those solutes which do not readily enter cells. A selective loss of water from the extracellular fluid compartment will raise its tonicity, causing osmotic water flow from cells (Fig. 3–3A). In consequence, the volume of the intracellular compartment will fall, thereby raising the intracellular solute concentration to equal that in the extracellular fluid. A selective gain of water by the extracellular fluid creates a relative

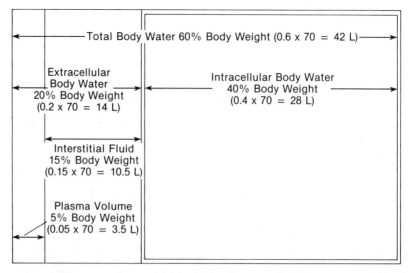

Figure 3–1. Schematic of normal body fluid volumes with representative values for a 70-kg person. (From Humes, H. D., Narins, R. G., and Brenner, B. M.: Disorders of water balance. Hosp. Prac. 14:133–145, 1979, with permission.)

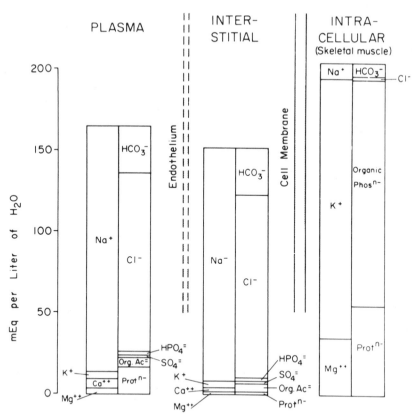

Figure 3–2. The major solute constituents of the main body fluid compartments. (Modified from Gamble, J. L.: Clinical Anatomy, Physiology, and Pathology of Extracellular Fluid. 6th Edition. Harvard University Press, 1954. From Valtin, H.: Renal Function: Mechanisms Preserving Fluid and Solute Balance in Health. 2nd Edition. Little, Brown & Co., Boston, 1983, with permission.)

hypertonicity in the intracellular compartment, promoting osmotic influx of water and thereby favoring osmotic equilibration across the cell membrane (Fig. 3–3B).

Osmolality differs from *tonicity* in that it is a measure of all of the dissolved species in an aqueous solution, not just those that fail to pass through cell membranes. For example, the osmolality (usually measured as change in freezing point or some other colligative property) of plasma with a high urea concentration will be elevated to above normal levels, assuming that the other usual solutes are at normal concentrations. However, because urea readily traverses cell membranes, it exerts no influence on the compartmental distribution of water or other solutes. Urea therefore influences the osmolality but not the tonicity of body fluids.

Fluid Movement Between Interstitial and Plasma Compartments. Fluid transfer between the plasma and the surrounding interstitial space occurs across the capillary walls. Capillaries, like cells, are freely permeable to water. Unlike cells, however, they also allow ready passage of salts, glucose, and other small molecules. Thus the ionic compositions of the interstitial and plasma fluids are much the same. Capillaries, however, limit the movement of plasma proteins. Therefore, the interstitial concentration of protein is much less than that of

Osmolality of extracellular fluid is determined by the concentration of all solutes, whereas tonicity is determined by the concentration of only those solutes unable to pass through cell membranes.

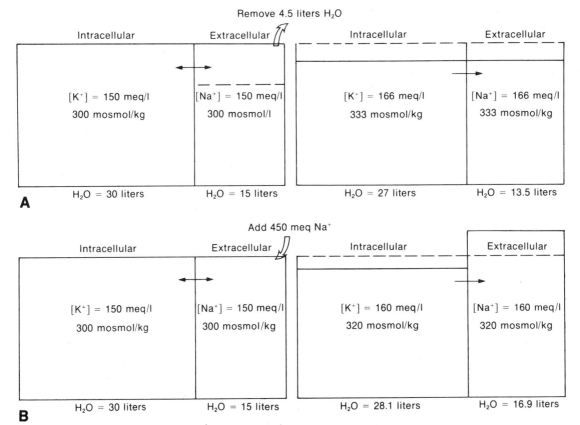

Figure 3–3. The response to changes in intra- and extracellular fluid volume are depicted schematically. (A) Removal of 4.5 liters of pure water from the extracellular compartment results in a redistribution of fluid and change in osmolality. (B) The effect of addition of 450 mEq of sodium to the extracellular fluid results in a different pattern of volume and osmolality redistribution. (From Aronson, P. S., and Thier, S. O.: The kidney. *In* Smith, L. H., and Thier, S. O., eds.: Pathophysiology. The Biologic Principles of Disease. 2nd Edition. W. B. Saunders Co., Philadelphia, 1985.)

plasma. This unequal distribution of protein generates an osmotic force often termed the *plasma oncotic pressure*. This osmotic force serves to pull fluid into capillaries, largely offsetting the outward movement of fluid driven by the *capillary hydraulic pressure*. The opposing effects of these two forces, the oncotic and hydraulic pressures, determine the distribution of fluid between the interstitial and plasma compartments. Clinical conditions in which plasma oncotic pressure is lowered (e.g., the hypoalbuminemia seen in protein malnutrition or nephrotic syndrome) will result in an imbalance of these capillary forces, favoring filtration of fluid into the interstitial space and the clinical appearance of edema. Similarly, if capillary hydraulic pressure rises as, for example, with venous occlusion, filtration of fluid will occur into the interstitial space and give rise to local edema formation.

HOMEOSTATIC RESPONSES TO ALTERED BODY FLUID TONICITY

The ability of all mammals to maintain body water content within narrow limits results from the interaction of three major physiologic effector mechanisms: (1) thirst and drinking; (2) stimulation or inhibition of ADH secretion; and (3) the ability of the kidneys to conserve or excrete water. (See Chapter 2 for a description of the renal concentrating-diluting mechanism.)

Thirst. Thirst, coupled with the physical ability to obtain water, is a primary defense of body fluid tonicity. Indeed, in the presence of a normal thirst mechanism and free access to water, plasma osmolality may be preserved at near-normal levels despite major defects in ADH release and/or the concentrating-diluting capacity of the kidney. While the cerebral cortex may influence drinking behavior, specific areas within the hypothalamus are critical to the regulation of water intake. Thirst is stimulated in these areas through an increase in the tonicity of body fluids, and inhibited by a reduction in tonicity. Also, isotonic reductions in extracellular volume are capable of enhancing thirst even without changes in tonicity. These stimuli are believed to be relayed by arterial and/or thoracic baroreceptors and subserve thirst control in circumstances such as hemorrhage or other alterations in cardiac output. In addition to these osmotic and nonosmotic (hemodynamic) stimuli, drinking is provoked by activation of the renin-angiotensin systems, probably via a direct dipsogenic effect of circulating angiotensin II on the hypothalamus. Indeed, angiotensin II is the most potent dipsogen studied to date. Pathologic derangements of thirst are rarely the sole cause of derangements of body fluid tonicity; however, in patients with acquired disturbances of serum tonicity regulation, abnormal drinking behavior often complicates defects in the other homeostatic control mechanisms.

Angiotensin II is the most powerful dipsogen known.

ADH Secretion. In hypothalamic centers adjacent to those controlling thirst, ADH is synthesized. From there ADH is transported to the posterior pituitary gland, from which it may be secreted into the circulation. Circulating ADH interacts with receptors in the terminal portions of the nephron (predominantly cortical and medullary collecting ducts), where it acts via adenylate cyclase to increase the permeability of these segments to water and thereby enhances urinary concentration and the conservation of water (see Chapter 2).

Changes in extracellular tonicity exert an important influence on hypothalamic synthesis and posterior pituitary release of ADH. Remarkably small elevations in plasma osmolality (as induced by water restriction) can induce several-fold increases of the circulating ADH level. An increment of plasma osmolality from a normal level of about 285 mOsm to one of 295 mOsm is capable of provoking a substantial increase in ADH secretion (Fig. 3–4). Moderate reductions of plasma osmolality suppress ADH to levels barely detectable even by sensitive radioimmunoassay. Although the primary function of ADH in states of water deficit and hypertonicity is to enhance collecting duct permeability to water, ADH, by virtue of its vasoconstrictive effects, also plays a role in regulating peripheral vascular resistance and systemic arterial blood pressure in circumstances of severe dehydration.

As with thirst, plasma osmolality is not the only factor that regulates ADH release. Several *non-osmotic factors* may also influence secretion of the hormone. Changes in extracellular fluid volume are important modulators of ADH release. Baroreceptors within the great vessels in the thorax presumably detect the pressure changes occasioned by alterations of the extracellular volume (?mechanical stretch) and these

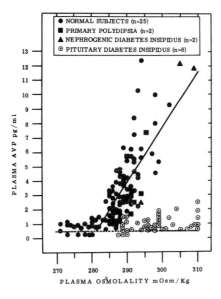

Figure 3–4. The relationship between plasma osmolality and plasma ADH (AVP) levels in normal subjects and in patients with polyuric disorders. AVP, arginine vasopressin. (From Robertson, G., et al.: Development and clinical application of a new method for the radioimmunoassay of arginine vasopressin in human plasma. J. Clin. Invest. 52:2340–2352, 1973, with permission of the American Society for Clinical Investigation.)

baroreceptors influence ADH release. In this way, reductions in extracellular volume provoke ADH secretion, whereas volume expansion suppresses secretion. Pain, other emotional stresses, and certain drugs (Table 3–1) also influence ADH release. Thus, non-osmotic stimuli to ADH secretion may lead to alterations in water excretion independent of disturbances in body fluid tonicity.

With failure of normal thirst, ADH secretion, and/or normal functioning of the renal concentrating mechanism, disturbances of hypo- and hypertonicity may ensue. In hypotonicity, serum osmolality and Na^+ concentration are low and clinical signs and symptoms of the hyponatremia are the result of cellular overhydration. When hypertonicity arises from failure of these control mechanisms, serum osmolality and Na^+ concentration are elevated and cells become dehydrated.

Na$^+$ concentration is the most important determinant of extracellular fluid tonicity.

HYPERTONIC STATES

Hypernatremia is the usual indication of hypertonicity since Na^+ is the dominant ion contributing to the tonicity of extracellular fluid. However, the increased serum Na^+ concentration implies nothing about the level of total body sodium. Total body sodium may be normal if hypertonicity is caused by pure water loss, whereas sodium stores may be diminished if some has been lost with a relatively greater loss

Table 3–1. DRUGS INFLUENCING ADH SECRETION

Stimulatory	Inhibitory
Narcotics	Ethanol
Tricyclic antidepressants	Narcotic antagonists
Cyclophosphamide	Phenytoin
Clofibrate	
Vincristine	
Nicotine	

of water. Occasionally total body sodium may be increased if Na$^+$ has been gained to a greater extent than water.

Distinguishing between the three possibilities of normal, low, and high total body sodium stores is a useful way of sorting the various diseases giving rise to hypernatremia (Fig. 3–5). While the patient's history may give some clue as to level of sodium balance, a more reliable assessment may be made by physical examination. Skin turgor, moisture of the mucous membranes, presence or absence of edema, the fullness of the jugular venous pulse, and postural changes in blood pressure and pulse are the indices used at the bedside to clarify the patient's level of total body sodium.

Hypernatremia Associated with Pure Water Loss. The lack of physical findings indicative of salt losses (dehydration and volume depletion) or excess (edema) implies a near-normal total body sodium content and, further, that the hypernatremia represents a loss of water alone. In this circumstance, substantial elevation of serum Na$^+$ concentration may occur with physiologically minor losses of plasma volume because such pure water losses are shared proportionally by both the intracellular and extracellular compartments. Since only about 8 percent of total body water is in the plasma compartment, even a large total water loss will inflict a relatively small loss of plasma volume. Hence, blood pressure and pulse are usually normal and tend not to change with position in the patient with pure water loss. For example, a 70-kg patient who loses about 5 liters of pure water will have lost only 400 ml from the plasma compartment, a volume which will not alter resting or postural blood pressure and pulse. However, such a loss will raise the serum Na$^+$ concentration to above 160 mEq/liter (Fig. 3–3A). Abnormalities of the clinical markers of plasma volume (thready pulse, tachycardia, orthostatic changes in pulse and blood pressure) in the hypernatremic patient usually imply that salt was lost with water or that truly massive losses of water have occurred. The signs associated with hypernatremia in the setting of normal total body sodium content are those of hypernatremia per se and consist mainly of generalized impairment of higher neurologic functions. The degree of neurologic impairment is roughly proportional to the degree of hypernatremia; symptoms are rarely present below a serum Na$^+$ concentration of 155 mEq/liter, whereas progressively more severe neurologic deficits occur beyond this level of hypernatremia.

Hypernatremia causes neurologic impairment to a degree proportional to the degree of hypernatremia present.

Hypodipsia. Primary isolated loss of thirst is a very rare cause of hypernatremia. However, more global neurologic dysfunction quite often provides the setting for hypernatremia, even with normal ADH secretion and normal renal water-conserving capacity. For example, some patients with extensive cerebral vascular disease may be unable to perceive thirst; others are just physically unable to get to water and to satisfy their perception of thirst. Such circumstances, added to normal ongoing insensible water losses of about 500 ml per day through respiration and evaporative dermal losses, will cause serum Na$^+$ concentration to rise. Increased water losses from hyperventilation, fever or sweating can accelerate this rise. Such neurologically impaired or severely disabled patients will have concentrated urine with osmolalities greater than 600 mOsm and variable amounts of sodium in the urine, largely reflecting their sodium intake. Treatment is with water

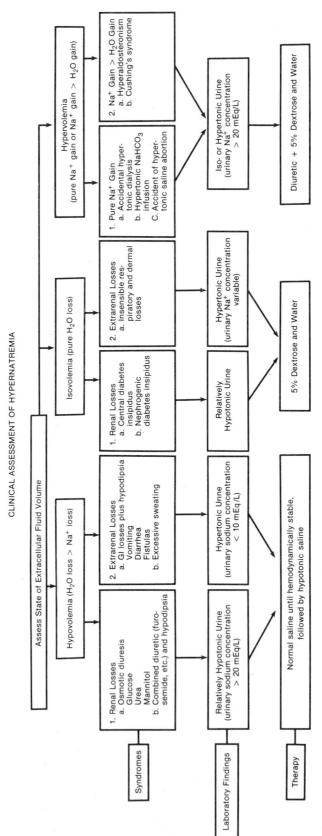

Figure 3–5. Categorization of hypernatremic disorders.

alone if a patient manifests pure water losses, i.e., has normal blood pressure and pulse. Usually, intravenous administration of 5 percent dextrose in water is effective. Calculations of water deficits are based on the following assumptions: (1) normal serum Na^+ is 140 mEq/liter; (2) total body water is 60 percent of body weight; and (3) body sodium acts as if it is distributed through total body water.

Example: What is the water deficit of a 70^g man with a serum Na^+ concentration of 154 mEq/liter?

Normal total body water: $70 \times 0.6 = 42$ liters

Normal total body sodium: 42 liters $\times$ 140 mEq/liter = 5,880 mEq

If it is assumed that total body sodium remains constant as water loss occurs, distribution of the same number of mEq of Na^+ in a lesser volume causes its concentration to increase to 154 mEq/liter.

$$\frac{5880 \text{ mEq}}{154 \text{ mEq/liter}} = 38.2 \text{ liters}$$

Thus, 3.8 liters $(42 - 38.2)$ of water were lost.

It should be noted that this calculation assumes pure water loss; to the degree that sodium has also been lost, the total fluid losses will be greater.

A set of defense mechanisms against cellular dehydration exists in brain cells. When dehydration is imposed, brain cells initially become dehydrated and shrink. with time, however, these cells return to their original volume despite continued dehydration and extracellular hypertonicity. The restoration of central nervous system volume results from an apparently unique ability of brain cells to generate within them so-called *idiogenic (unidentified) osmoles,* which serve to draw water into cells and restore cell volume. Because of the production within brain cells of these osmotically active substances during chronic hypernatremia, restdoration of the calculated water deficit must proceed gradually. Rapid administration of water before dissipation of these intraneural substances may lead to brain edema and even death. To avoid this complication the rate of fluid administration should be timed to lower serum osmolality by no more than 2 mOsm per hour, with serum Na^+ concentration decreasing by no more than 1 mEq per hour. To ensure this rate of decline, serum electrolyte levels must be monitored at frequent intervals.

Rehydration of a hypernatremic patient can be fatal if serum electrolyte monitoring is not done carefully.

Diabetes Insipidus. *Clinical Aspects and Classification.* Diabetes insipidus (DI) may be caused by failure of the hypothalamic synthesis of ADH (central, pituitary, or neurogenic DI) or a failure of the kidney to respond to ADH which is synthesized and released normally (nephrogenic DI) (Figs. 3–4 and 3–6). In either case polyuria ensues and urine osmolality is equal to or less than plasma. Since these defects in ADH secretion or action entail no necessary losses of Na^+, Na^+ excretion usually matches dietary intake. Thus, the abnormal losses are essentially those of pure water.

In cases of nephrogenic or central DI, the daily urinary losses may be extraordinary, ranging up to 20 liters per day. However, severe hypertonicity and hypernatremia rarely supervene even in such extreme cases and only occur when the ability to acquire water is

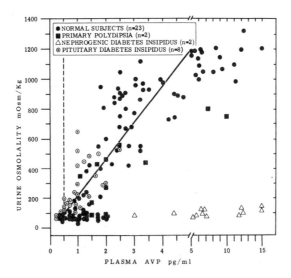

Figure 3–6. The relationship between plasma ADH (AVP) and urine osmolality in normal subjects and in patients with polyuric disorders. (From Robertson, G., et al.: Development and clinical application of a new method for the radio-immunoassay of arginine vasopressin in human plasma. J. Clin. Invest. 52:2340–2352, 1973, with permission.)

compromised. Thus, in the presence of a normal thirst mechanism and the ability to drink, patients with DI are polyuric but not more than mildly hypertonic. Obviously, even transient neurologic disturbances or lack of access to water will lead quickly to hypernatremia in such patients.

A number of central nervous system disorders may produce central DI (Table 3–2). the most common specific causes are surgery, trauma, and tuumors; infectious and vascular diseases are far less commonly involved. As many as 50 percent of cases have no discernible cause.

Congenital nephrogenic diabetes insipidus is a rare hereditary disorder resulting from renal tubules insensitivity to ADH (Fig. 3–6). The disease is more severe in males and appears to have a sex-linked dominant inheritance. It presents in early childhood with dehydration and an inability to concentrate the urine.

A wide variety of acquired or congenital disorders, drugs, or electrolyte and nutritional imbalances can alter the kidney's ability to concentrate urine.

Cases of *acquired nephrogenic DI* for outnumber those of cental DI or congenital nephrogenic DI. Generally, acquired nephrogenic DI precipitates complaints of nocturia/more often than frank polyuria. In keeping with the lesser daily urine volume, dehydration, hypertonicity, and hypernatremia are unusual occurrences. However, if consciousness is impaired or access to water is limited, the mild-to-moderate polyuria may result in overt dehydration. A large variety of acquired disorders may diminish the kidney's ability to maximally concentrate the urine

Table 3–2. ETIOLOGIC FACTORS IN CENTRAL (NEUROGENIC) DIABETES INSIPIDUS

Posthypophysectomy
Idiopathic (including familial forms)
Post-traumatic
Hypothalamic and pituitary tumors (metastatic, craniopharyngioma, etc.)
Cysts
Histiocytosis
Granuloma (tuberculosis, sarcoidosis)
Vascular abnormalities (aneurysm, thrombosis, Sheehan's syndrome)
Infections (meningitis, encephalitis)

Table 3–3. ETIOLOGIC FACTORS IN NEPHROGENIC DIABETES INSIPIDUS

Congenital nephrogenic DI
Acquired nephrogenic DI
    Chronic renal disease
    Urinary tract obstruction
    Analgesic nephropathy
    Pyelonephritis
    Polycystic kidney disease
    Multiple myeloma
    Amyloidosis
    Hypercalcemia
    Hypokalemia
    Sjögren's syndrome
    Sickle cell anemia
    Drugs (lithium, methoxyflurane, demeclocycline, amphotericin B)

(Table 3–3). Virtually any intrinsic renal disease that substantially reduces the glomerular filtration rate will be accompanied by some degree of nephrogenic DI, as defined by the inability to maximally concentrate urine. Additionally, several electrolyte and nutritional disorders as well as some drugs can diminish concentrating capacity. Chronic intrinsic renal diseases disturb the concentrating mechanism through several means. Those diseases that preferentially destroy the renal medulla such as obstructive uropathy, sickle cell disease, and analgesic nephropathy are particularly likely to induce nephrogenic DI. Diseases afflicting the glomeruli and the tubulointerstitial compartment limit urinary concentration by at least two mechanisms in addition to direct medullary damage. First, the osmotic load per surviving nephron is increased because of the elevated level of filtered urea and the increased glomerular filtration rate of surviving nephrons. In this way an osmotic diuresis is imposed on residual nephrons. Second, a cellular resistance to ADH develops in the collecting ducts of the surviving nephrons. The precise cellular defect has yet to be identified; however, a failure of ADH to generate cyclic AMP in this nephron segment does not appear to explain this ADH resistance since cyclic AMP analogues also fail to enhance the water permeability of the terminal nephron of uremic animals.

Severe limitations of dietary protein will also reduce the ability to concentrate urine because of the reduced availability of urea, which provides about one half of medullary interstitial hypertonicity. Since it is this hypertonicity that constitutes the osmotic gradient for water reabsorption across the collecting duct, a fall in the urea concentration of the medulla reduces water reabsorption and urine concentration (see Chapter 2). Sodium depletion may also reduce maximal urine concentration. Presumably in such a circumstance, enhanced proximal reabsorption of sodium results in less salt delivered to the ascending limb where active and passive transport mechanisms serve to transfer NaCl to the medullary interstitium. Thus, the tonicity of the medullary interstitium is diminished and a concentrating deficit is established.

Hypercalcemia and *hypokalemia* are the most notable abnormalities of serum electrolytes that lead to nephrogenic DI. The mechanism by which hypercalcemia interferes with concentration of the urine is not entirely clear but probably involves both a reduction in medullary tonicity (caused by suppression of Na^+ reabsorption in the ascending limb) and an antagonistic effect on the influence of ADH on the collecting duct. Hypokalemia causes polyuria by enhancing thirst but also by interfering with the renal concentrating mechanism, perhaps by enhancing renal medullary prostaglandin synthesis and thereby causing enhanced washout of medullary interstitial hypertonicity.

Lithium carbonate, employed to treat manic-depressive disorders, often causes polyuria though usually not of disabling degree. Medullary tonicity appears to be preserved and the abnormality involves a reduced responsiveness of the terminal nephron to ADH. Additional drugs that may induce concentrating defects include amphotericin B, demeclocycline, and methoxyflurane.

Diagnosis. Central DI should be considered as a cause for polyuria, particularly when the symptom appears suddenly. Nephrogenic DI usually has a more gradual onset and also is rarely associated with more than 5 liters of urine per day. In addition to central DI, two other major causes of polyuria with an abrupt onset must be considered (Fig. 3–7). First, osmotic diuresis is generally noted by the presence of glycosuria; however, solutes other than glucose may occasionally be present in sufficient quantities to produce an osmotic diuresis. For example, high protein feeding may evoke urea-induced osmotic diuresis. Measurement of the rate of osmolar excretion over a brief period will identify the patient with an osmotic diuresis (Fig. 3–8). If osmolar excretion exceeds 50 mOsm/hr (normal rates are about 25 mOsm/hr), an osmotic diuresis is the likely cause of the polyuria. The other major consideration in cases of polyuria is *primary or psychogenic polydipsia*. While such patients are never hypertonic (indeed, their plasma osmolalities tend to be slightly below normal), they elaborate a large volume of hypotonic urine and in this regard mimic the patient with central DI.

In the absence of readily available measurements of plasma ADH levels, several protocols for stimulating ADH release have been devised to distinguish between central DI, nephrogenic DI, and primary polydipsia. Fluid deprivation remains the standard method for differentiating those disorders (Fig. 3–8). The patient is deprived of fluid

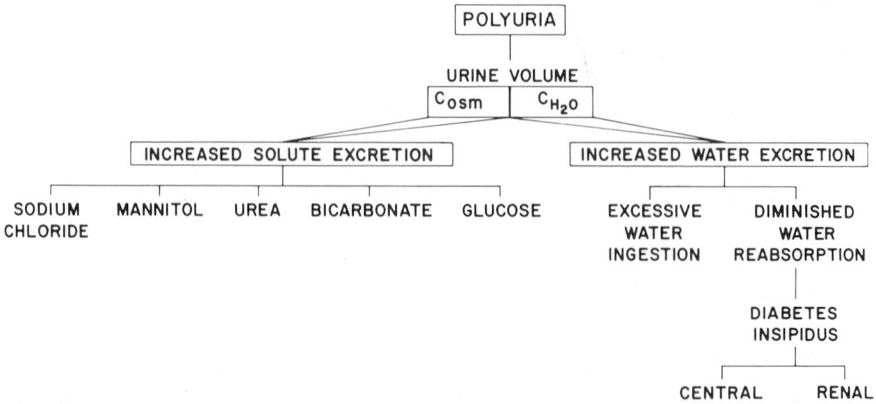

Abrupt-onset polyuria is most often caused by central diabetes insipidus, osmotic diuresis, or psychogenic polydipsia.

Figure 3–7. The multiple causes of polyuria. (Courtesy of Dr. R. G. Narins.)

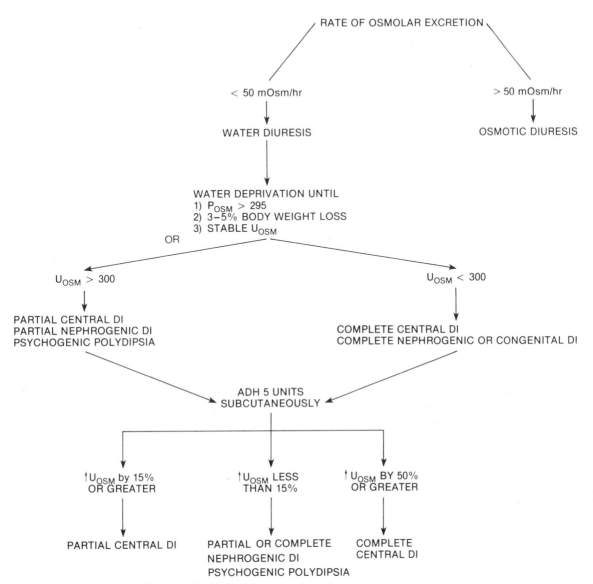

Figure 3–8. Diagnostic approach to the patient with polyuria.

until any of the following end points is reached: plasma osmolality exceeds 295 mOsm, body weight falls by 3 to 5 percent, or three consecutive hourly urine samples demonstrate a plateau in urine osmolality. Reaching these points ordinarily requires 12 to 16 hours of fluid restriction, during which time the patient's cardiovascular status must be followed closely to avoid harmful dehydration in the patient with complete DI. If, when such a degree of dehydration is achieved, the patient's urine osmolality remains less than that of plasma, the patient has either complete central DI, the less common congenital nephrogenic DI, or the least common, severe acquired nephrogenic DI.

Central DI may be distinguished from nephrogenic DI by the urinary response to exogenous ADH (5 U of aqueous ADH injected·

subcutaneously). Patients with central DI will develop an increase in urine osmolality of 50 percent or more within one to two hours, while patients with nephrogenic DI will display little or no increase in urine osmolality. If, at the point of dehydration, the patient's urine osmolality exceeds that of plasma, the patient has either partial DI (central or nephrogenic) or psychogenic polydipsia. Generally, the urine osmolality of patients with all three of these partial disorders will be greater than the osmolality of plasma but less than the maximal value found in normal dehydrated subjects (1000 to 1200 mOsm).

The response to exogenous ADH by patients in these three categories further subdivides them. Those with partial central DI will augment their urine osmolalities, while those with partial nephrogenic DI or primary polydipsia show little or no response. Patients with primary polydipsia fail to develop maximal urinary osmolalities with this degree of dehydration and exogenous ADH because of the dissipation or "washout" of the renal medullary hypertonicity by prolonged self-imposed water diuresis. However, if physiologically appropriate water intake can be maintained in such patients, they regain the ability to maximally concentrate their urine.

With the availability of radioimmunoassay measurements of ADH levels in plasma, the categorization of these disorders has become somewhat simpler (Figs. 3–4 and 3–6). With dehydration, plasma ADH levels remain low in patients with central DI, and high (but equal to dehydrated normal subjects) in patients with nephrogenic DI and primary polydipsia. The latter remains a diagnosis suggested by low plasma osmolalities before dehydrating maneuvers and by a history of abnormal behavior.

Therapy. Nephrogenic DI is most effectively treated where possible by correcting the underlying disorder, such as hypokalemia or hypercalcemia. Although many categories of nephrogenic DI result from fixed structural lesions of the renal medulla and papilla (amyloidosis, polycystic kidney disease), most patients with these forms do not require treatment since polyuria tends to be mild. However, patients with congenital nephrogenic DI and occasional patients with the acquired form will exhibit more marked polyuria and therefore require therapy. The standard mode of therapy is the combination of a *low-salt diet* and *thiazide diuretics*. This regimen lowers the urine flow rate by several mechanisms. The initial negative Na^+ balance induced by the diuretic leads to reduced delivery of filtrate into the defective concentrating apparatus in the renal medulla (limbs of Henle and medullary collecting ducts). This may be caused by reduced glomerular filtration or, more likely, enhanced proximal tubule fluid reabsorption, both consequences of the negative Na^+ balance and plasma volume contraction. Of interest, preliminary evidence suggests that prostaglandin synthesis inhibitors may be useful adjuncts to thiazides and low-salt diet. Both indomethacin and ibuprofen were capable of enhancing the antidiuretic acitvity of a thiazide in two patients with presumably congenital nephrogenic DI. Recent basic research provides ample rationale for such therapy in that prostaglandins appear to be synthesized in ADH-responsive epithelia and function as local counter-regulators of ADH action by opposing the peptide hormone's effect on collecting duct water permeability. The role of inhibitors of prostaglan-

Standard therapy for congenital nephrogenic diabetes insipidus is low-salt diet and thiazide diuretics.

din production in the therapy of nephrogenic DI remains to be further defined in a larger group of patients including those with acquired forms of the disorder.

Chronic therapy of complete central DI centers on *exogenous ADH* replacement. The analogue, desmopressin acetate (DDAVP), is the drug of choice and is administered as a nasal spray one to four times daily. Vasopressin tannate in oil can be administered once daily with equally good control of urine flow but requires intramuscular injection. Acute therapy in patients unable to use nasal sprays should consist of aqueous vasopressin and adequate replacement of water deficits.

Complete central DI therapy:
● *desmopressin acetate*
● *vasopressin tannate*
Partial central DI therapy:
● *chlorpropamide*
● *clofibrate*

Partial forms of central DI may be controlled with *chlorpropamide.* This oral hypoglycemic agent appears to exert its beneficial effects by suppressing prostaglandin synthesis and thereby reducing their antagonism of the small amounts of ADH present in plasma. The drug probably does not affect ADH secretion; rather, it appears to enhance the action of ADH. Hypoglycemia is, of course, a potential side effect of chlorpropamide. Two other drugs have had success in some patients with partial congenital DI. *Clofibrate* seems to enhance ADH release, though plasma levels of ADH before and after administration of this drug have not yet been reported. Carbamazepine may also be useful; however, its mode of action is uncertain since reports of its effects on ADH secretion are conflicting.

Hypernatremia Associated with Combined Sodium and Water Losses. Three sources of losses may give rise to hypertonicity in the presence of perceptible Na^+ deficits (see Fig. 3–5). Fluids lost from kidney, gastrointestinal tract, and skin are generally low in Na^+ concentration, so in themselves such losses of relatively more water than solute tend to raise serum Na^+ concentration. However, normal thirst mechanisms drive the usual patient with such losses to drink more water. Thus, as with the pure water losses described above, hypernatremia in this setting implies a failure of thirst, or such physical incapacity that water cannot be acquired.

Non-renal losses through diarrhea, vomiting, or excess sweating include appreciable amounts of Na^+ so that the usual clinical evidences of plasma volume depletion, tachycardia, hypotension, or postural provocation of these signs, are often present. Also, the kidney responds appropriately to the salt and water deficits and so urine osmolality is typically high (>800 mOsm) and urine Na^+ concentration low (<10 mEq/liter). These urine values differ from those seen when renal losses are the genesis of the volume depletion and hypertonicity, in which case urine tends to be nearly isotonic with plasma, and urine Na^+ concentrations are relatively high (>20 mEq/liter).

Such hypotonic renal losses derive from either osmotic diuresis or drug-induced diuresis and natriuresis. Osmotic diuresis occurs when the concentration of a solute in the glomerular filtrate exceeds the reabsorptive capacity of the renal tubules. The residuum of unreabsorbed solute obligates the retention of water within the tubule and an increased amount of fluid with a low salt concentration is delivered distally. Because of the increased delivery of a fluid with a lower NaCl content, the ability of the thick ascending limb of Henle to actively generate a gradient of NaCl is overwhelmed and the development of the interstitial hypertonicity necessary for maximal urinary concentration is blunted. As indicated in Figure 3–7, *glucose* is the most common solute to lead to this series of events, as in poorly controlled diabetes mellitus. Occasionally, protein ingestion or amino acid infusions may cause sufficient urea production to generate a strong *urea diuresis*. *Mannitol*, usually administered to reduce cerebral edema, of course generates an osmotic diuresis and, as with glucose or urea, hypertonicity may ensue. Infusions of hypertonic NaCl or $NaHCO_3$ may also induce osmotic diuresis in some patients given excessively large quantities of these solutes.

Recognition of hypernatremia associated with Na^+ losses mandates treatment by first attempting to stem the particular loss and replacing deficits accordingly. Cardiovascular compromise with hypotension demands initial treatment with isotonic NaCl and/or colloid volume expanders. Once arterial blood pressure and pulse have been restored to the normal range with this maneuver, correction of the serum tonicity can be pursued as outlined for pure water losses, that is, slow infusion of hypotonic fluids to avoid cerebral edema.

Hypernatremia Associated with Sodium Gain. Hypernatremia resulting from sodium gain is seen far less frequently than either the pure water losses or the hypotonic losses with sodium depletion. Patients with *primary aldosteronism* tend to develop mild hypernatremia, with serum Na^+ concentrations rising to 150–155 mEq/liter. This slight elevation of Na^+ concentration is thought to arise by two mechanisms. First, aldosterone enhances Na^+ reabsorption in the distal nephron at sites where a proportionally smaller amount of water is reabsorbed so that more Na^+ than water is returned to the circulation. Second, the resulting extracellular volume expansion suppresses the renin-angiotensin and ADH systems, removing these dipsogenic and water-retentive forces. Thus, such patients persist with mild hypernatremia.

More severe degrees of hypernatremia with Na^+ overload occur with the acute addition of hypertonic NaCl or $NaHCO_3$ to the extracellular fluid. Water is withdrawn from cells and acute expansion of the extracellular volume and dilution of plasma proteins may lead to acute pulmonary edema. Moreover, the suddenness of the hypernatremia precludes the cerebral production of idiogenic osmoles. Therefore, the brain, like other tissues, is forced to give up intracellular water and the resulting shrinkage predisposes to intracranial hemorrhage or other potentially serious neurological deficits. This catastrophic series of events is rare and most often iatrogenic. Rapid administration of standard $NaHCO_3$ solutions (whose osmolality is approximately 800 mOsm) is the most common cause, as during attempts at cardiac resuscitation. Other circumstances include accidental administration of hypertonic NaCl, errors in mixing of dialysis solutions, and accidental substitution of salt for sugar in feeding formulas.

Therapy is directed at removing the excess salt with potent diuretics, and quantitative replacement of the urinary losses of water with intravenous 5 percent dextrose solution. Oliguric patients with sodium overload may require dialysis to correct hypertonicity and volume expansion.

HYPOTONIC STATES

Hypotonicity of the body fluids is most often recognized by the finding of hyponatremia. However, it is important to realize that while all hypotonic patients are hyponatremic, not all hyponatremic patients are hypotonic. Measurement of the serum osmolality distinguishes hypotonic hyponatremia from the isotonic and hypertonic varieties (Fig. 3–9 and Table 3–4).

Isotonic Hyponatremia. *Isotonic hyponatremia,* sometimes termed "pseudohyponatremia," occurs when abnormal proteins or excessive lipids appear in the serum. The two most common conditions giving rise to these findings are multiple myeloma and hyperlipidemia. Low serum Na^+ concentrations are obtained because of the increase in the volume of the solid components in the serum contributed by the excess protein or lipid (normally such substances account for only about 6 to 8 percent of the volume of serum). Thus, in a given aliquot of serum

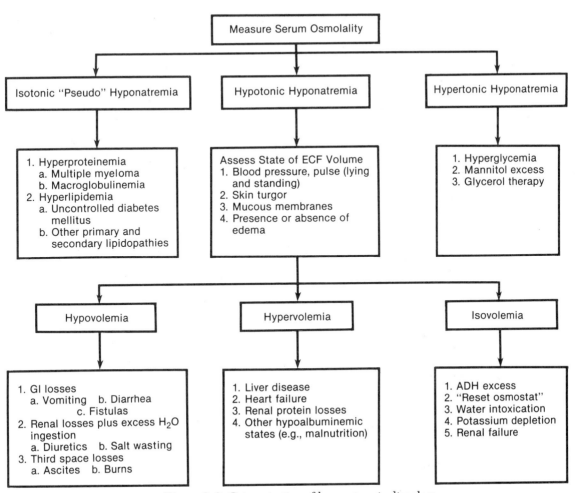

Figure 3–9. Categorization of hyponatremic disorders.

Table 3–4. LABORATORY DIAGNOSIS OF THE HYPONATREMIAS

	Serum					Urine		
						Osmolality		
	BUN	Uric Acid	Lipids	Total Protein	Glucose	Basal	After Water Load	Sodium (mEq/L)
Isotonic Hyponatremia								
Hyperlipidemia	N	N, ↑	↑↑	N	N	Variable	Dilute	Variable
Hyperproteinemia	N	N	N	↑↑	N	Variable	Dilute	Variable
Hypertonic Hyponatremia								
Hyperglycemia	N, ↑	N	N, ↑	N	↑↑	Isotonic		> 20
Mannitol excess	N, ↑	N	N	N	N	Isotonic		> 20
Hypotonic Hyponatremia								
ECF Volume Depleted								
GI fluid loss or third space loss	↑↑	N, ↑	N	N, ↑	N	Hypertonic	IH	< 20
Renal (adrenal) loss	↑	N, ↑	N	N, ↑	N	Isotonic ± Hypertonic	IH	> 20
ECF Volume Expanded	N, ↑	N, ↑	N	N	N	IH	IH	< 20
ECF Volume "Normal"								
SIADH	N, ↓	N, ↓	N	N, ↓	N	IH	IH	Reflects diet
"Reset osmostat"	N, ↓	N	N	N	N	IH	Dilute	> 20

Serum Osmolality Normal or Elevated *(Isotonic and Hypertonic Hyponatremia)*
Serum Osmolality Low *(Hypotonic Hyponatremia)*

N = Normal   IH = Inappropriately hypertonic   ↑ = Minor elevation   ↑↑ = Major elevation   ↓ = Minor reduction the volume attributable to water (normally about 93 percent) will be diminished. Since the Na^+ is distributed only in the aqueous phase, the amount of Na^+ in that aliquot of serum will be less and a reduced serum Na^+ concentration will be measured (Table 3–4). However, the osmolality of the serum will remain normal because the usual tests of osmolality rely only on the activity of the solutes in aqueous phase. Most importantly, patients with isotonic hyponatremia incur none of the ill effects of hypotonic hyponatremia. Thus, no treatment need be directed toward this form of hyponatremia per se, but of course analysis and therapy of the abnormality of serum proteins or lipids is required.

Hypertonic Hyponatremia. Hypertonicity may also accompany hyponatremia. The addition to the extracellular fluid of a solute which is impermeant to cells will cause water to move out of the intracellular space and into the extracellular compartment, thereby diluting all the solutes in the extracellular fluid, including Na^+. Diabetic hyperglycemia and the therapeutic administration of mannitol or glycerol are the usual clinical situations in which hypertonic hyponatremia appears (Table 3–4). The presence of hypertonicity despite hyponatremia is established by measurement of the serum osmolality, which is high.

An approximation of the serum osmolality can be obtained from the routine measurements of serum Na^+, glucose, and blood urea nitrogen (BUN) concentrations by the following equation:

Calculated osmolality =

$$2Na(mEq/liter) + \frac{glucose\ (mg/dl)}{18} + \frac{BUN\ (mg/dl)}{2.8}$$

The sodium concentration is multiplied by two to account for its attendant monovalent anions, Cl^- or HCO_3^-. Because glucose and BUN are conventionally expressed in mg/0.1 liter (dl), they are divided by 1/10 of their molecular weights. The calculated osmolality is usually within 10 to 15 mOsm of the measured value. If the measured osmolality exceeds the calculated value by more than this margin, then an unmeasured solute such as mannitol is present.

Blood urea nitrogen (BUN) is increased by infection, postoperative catabolism, postpartum involution, and administration of catabolic drugs such as adrenal steroids and tetracycline.

Hypotonic Hyponatremia. Hypotonic hyponatremia is the most common form of hyponatremia (Fig. 3–9 and Table 3–4). Neurologic abnormalities resulting from the low extracellular fluid osmolality may be nonspecific and range from lethargy and mild changes in sensorium to seizures and coma. The degree of central nervous system dysfunction is related to the level of hyponatremia; only minor disturbances are usually noted when serum Na^+ concentration is above 120 mEq/liter; more serious abnormalities are common below 115 mEq/liter. The presence or absence of neurologic signs may be influenced by many factors including the rate at which hyponatremia develops, with greater abnormalities seen after more rapid falls in serum Na^+ concentration.

As with hypernatremia, it is useful to further subdivide hypotonic hyponatremia according to the patient's total body sodium stores (Fig. 3–9). Again the serum Na^+ concentration implies nothing about the patient's total body sodium content and the status of the latter is determined at the bedside from such indices as skin turgor, moisture of mucous membranes, and orthostatic changes in blood pressure or pulse.

Hyponatremia Associated with Combined Sodium and Water Losses. Extracellular volume depletion frequently is associated with hyponatremia. In such hypovolemic states, the homeostatic mechanisms that contribute to maintenance of an adequate circulating blood volume appear to supersede those maintaining body fluid tonicity. Thus, ADH secretion is stimulated by the non-osmotic signals arising from the recognition of extracellular volume contraction and leads to ongoing renal water retention despite hyponatremia and hypotonicity.

Besides the ADH-induced increase in terminal nephron permeability to water, volume contraction promotes increased fluid reabsorption in the proximal tubule and may reduce glomerular filtration rate as well. These latter effects lead to decreased delivery of fluid to the distal diluting segments and, while conserving fluid further, limit the capacity to generate and excrete the dilute urine necessary for repair of the hypotonic state.

As already noted, fluid losses from the kidney, skin, and gastrointestinal tract tend to be hypotonic and in themselves lead to hypertonicity and volume depletion. The hyponatremia which follows these abnormal losses must therefore be generated by the patient's ingestion (or physician's administration) of excessive quantities of water as replacement for the losses of hypotonic body fluids. The hyponatremia is then maintained by the altered renal handling of water outlined above.

Deficits of fluid arising from skin or gastrointestinal losses (or internal sequestration) are met by the renal conservation of salt and water so that urinary osmolality tends to be high and Na^+ concentration low (<10 mEq/liter). In several circumstances, however, the kidney itself may be the route of inordinate volume loss. Patients with chronic renal insufficiency manifest a sluggish renal response to extracellular volume contraction so that maximal urinary conservation of salt and water is blunted. Thus, extrarenal losses may not be readily checked in such patients and the diseased kidney will play a supporting role in the generation of volume contraction. Primary renal losses of salt and water exceeding usual daily intakes are rarely caused by intrinsic renal disease. However, a variety of tubulointerstitial diseases and particularly chronic obstruction and medullary cystic disease may occasionally lead to *salt wasting*.

"Salt wasting," the primary renal loss of salt and water exceeding daily intake, often results from chronic obstruction or medullary cystic disease.

Adrenal insufficiency is classically associated with hypotonic hyponatremia and extracellular volume contraction. ADH levels are high in experimental and clinical adrenal insufficiency. Mineralocorticoid deficiency and extracellular volume contraction from renal salt losses do not appear, however, to entirely explain the stimulation of ADH secretion. The absence of glucocorticoids leads to reduced cardiac output which serves as an additional stimulus to ADH release. Glucocorticoid deficiency per se has also been found to enhance distal permeability to water. Thus, the defect in water excretion in the addisonian patient is probably multifactorial.

Diuretic-induced fluid losses, whether from osmotic agents or natriuretic drugs, are typically associated with volume depletion and enhanced ADH secretion. The volume contraction may also reduce glomerular filtration rate and promote proximal fluid reabsorption, effects which reduce delivery to the loop of Henle. Also, thiazides, furosemide, and ethacrynic acid inhibit the active reabsorption of salt in the diluting segment and therefore reduce the capacity to generate dilute urine. Finally, the K^+ losses in many of these patients may allow movement of Na^+ into cells, contributing further to the severity of hyponatremia.

Treatment of the hyponatremia associated with renal and nonrenal losses of salt can be effectively achieved by restoration of the extracellular volume. Infusion of isotonic saline or colloid-containing solutions is the first step in circumstances of severe hypotension. Diuretic use should, of course, be discontinued and more specific therapy, such as replacement of adrenal steroids, may be indicated.

Hyponatremia Associated with Edema. Patients with hypotonic hyponatremia may also present at the other extreme of total body sodium stores, that is, with expansion of extracellular volume (Fig. 3–9 and Table 3–4). This general category is defined by the presence of peripheral edema and/or ascites. Conventionally, patients with congestive heart failure and cirrhosis are conceived as having a reduced "effective" arterial blood volume. In the case of heart failure, the reduced cardiac output is the primary hemodynamic abnormality which activates salt- and water-conserving mechanisms both within and outside the kidney. Similarly, the reduced peripheral vascular resistance, enlargement of the splanchnic bed, and formation of ascitic fluid are the means by which the cardiac output is rendered relatively ineffective in cirrhosis and similar salt- and water-retentive mechanisms are activated.

Enhanced release of ADH appears to be common to both cirrhosis and heart failure. The higher circulating levels of this hormone represent one of the reasons for impaired water excretion in these patients. In addition, the lower glomerular filtration rate and increased proximal fluid reabsorption conspire to further diminish diluting capability. Finally, administration of thiazide or loop diuretics to these patients may add another impediment to their already impaired renal diluting capacity. Thus, with this combination of insults to solute-free water generation and excretion, ingestion of even modest amounts of water may prove excessive and lead to hyponatremia. Unless diuretics have been given to these patients, their urine usually demonstrates a low Na^+ concentration and relatively high osmolality, evidence of avid renal conservation of salt and water (Table 3–4).

Advanced renal failure may be the setting for hypotonic hyponatremia associated with volume overload. In a patient with a glomerular filtration rate of only 5 to 10 ml/min (about 7 to 14 liters/day), the delivery of fluid into the nephron and, more important, the loop and distal diluting segments becomes so limited that relatively moderate increments in water intake cannot be excreted. Thus, unlike the individual with normal renal function, these patients may become hyponatremic with ingestion or infusion of only a few extra liters of water. Urine Na^+ concentration will generally be high in such patients and reflect their dietary sodium intake, while urine osmolality will be very nearly isotonic to plasma (Table 3–4).

Although the renal and extrarenal mechanisms for limiting water excretion are similar in edematous and volume-depleted states (reduced glomerular filtration rate, enhanced proximal fluid reabsorption, and augmented ADH release), the therapies are obviously different. Volume expansion is the appropriate reply to volume contraction, whereas volume expansion would be inappropriate and even life-threatening in the already edematous patient. In edematous patients, efforts to improve the underlying condition must be attempted. However, such specific therapy is usually insufficient to rectify fully the underlying heart failure or cirrhosis. For this reason, fluid restriction becomes the major means for raising the serum sodium concentration in these cases.

Hyponatremia Associated with Near-Normal Extracellular Volume. Syndrome of Inappropriate ADH Secretion. A large group of patients displaying hypotonic hyponatremia appear to have normal total body sodium stores (isovolemia) as judged by the usual bedside criteria (Fig. 3–9). The syndrome of inappropriate secretion of ADH (SIADH) includes many of these cases (Table 3–5). In these patients ADH release occurs in the face of hypotonicity and normal-to-mildly elevated total body water (Fig. 3–10). Thus, the secretion of ADH is inappropriate to the known prevailing major osmotic and non-osmotic stimuli. Pain and other emotional stresses may account for the ADH release in certain patients, while in others the administration of a drug such as a *narcotic* or *barbiturate* (Table 3–1) stimulates ADH release. Finally, a large fraction of patients with elevated ADH levels in this setting have *central nervous system diseases, pulmonary diseases* or an *ADH-secreting tumor* (Table 3–5). It is to this last group that the term SIADH is most often applied. Brain disorders and head trauma may allow ADH release from the hypothalamus and/or pituitary in an unstimulated and osmotically unregulated fashion. Ectopic ADH may be produced from several malignancies, most notably oat cell carcinoma of the lung; early studies discovered ADH-like material in lung tissue from patients with pulmonary infections. Regardless of the source, the elevated hormone levels limit water excretion by enhancing water reabsorption from the collecting ducts so that ingested water is retained.

The syndrome of inappropriate ADH secretion (SIADH) is most often caused by an ADH-secreting tumor.

Table 3–5. DISORDERS ASSOCIATED WITH SIADH

Malignant tumors	Pulmonary diseases *Continued*
Lung (oat cell)	Cystic fibrosis
Pancreas	Asthma
Duodenum	Positive pressure ventilation
Urinary bladder	Drugs
Prostate	Vasopressin
Lymphoma	Oxytocin
Central nervous system disorders	Vincristine
Meningitis, encephalitis	Vinblastine
Head trauma	Phenothiazine
Brain tumor or abscess	Carbamazepine
Guillain-Barré syndrome	Clofibrate
Acute intermittent porphyria	Nicotine
Subarachnoid hemorrhage	Acute psychosis
Hydrocephalus	
Delirium tremens	Postoperative state
Pulmonary diseases	Myxedema
Pneumonia	"Reset osmostat"
Tuberculosis	
Lung abscess	"Idiopathic"

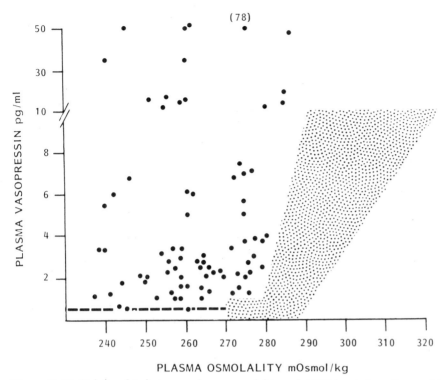

Figure 3–10. Relationship between plasma osmolality and ADH levels in patients with SIADH. Shaded area denotes normal range. Plasma vasopressin levels in patients with SIADH are inappropriately elevated for their state of reduced plasma osmolality. (From Zerbe, R., Stropes, L., and Robertson, G.: Vasopressin function in the syndrome of inappropriate antidiuresis. Ann. Rev. Med. 31:315–327, 1980, with permission.)

The retention of fluid is eventually limited by other overriding mechanisms (see Chapter 2) so that clinically apparent increments of body fluid volumes are not attained. After the gain of about 2 kg of fluid, subjects infused with exogenous ADH come into balance and begin to excrete essentially the amount of water and salt they ingest. Thus, urinary Na^+ excretion typically matches dietary intake and therefore the urine Na^+ concentration is usually greater than 20 mEq/liter (Table 3–4). This persistent excretion of a relative Na^+-rich urine, along with the water retention, contributes to the hyponatremia of SIADH. However, urine osmolalities remain inappropriately elevated, given the low extracellular fluid tonicity.

The mild, clinically imperceptible volume expansion in such patients with normal kidneys leads to the increased clearance of nitrogenous wastes, notably urea and uric acid. For this reason, BUN and serum uric acid levels tend to be reduced in SIADH and these laboratory findings may be a useful clue to separating hyponatremic patients with SIADH from those with volume depletion or edema discussed above, in whom BUN and uric acid levels are usually elevated (Table 3–4).

The treatment of the hypotonic hyponatremia associated with SIADH depends largely on the clinical status of the patient. Asymptomatic patients should be treated conservatively with water restriction and careful observation. Symptomatic patients require more vigorous therapy. While the degree of symptoms is generally related to the level of serum Na^+ concentration (and osmolality), occasional patients with levels of 120 mEq/liter (and similarly low plasma osmolalities) or even below may be remarkably asymptomatic, presumably because of the slow development of the hypotonic state. Although such hyponatremia requires treatment, this can usually be effected on a non-urgent basis. On the other hand, the hypotonic hyponatremic patient with more than minor changes in sensorium requires aggressive therapy. Infusion of hypertonic saline may correct the hyponatremia; however, in the presence of pre-existing mild volume expansion from water retention, the risk of pulmonary edema may be considerable. By inducing a diuresis with furosemide and quantitatively replacing the hypotonic urinary sodium losses with isotonic saline, the risk is largely obviated.

Chronic correction of SIADH is often achieved just by water restriction alone. In those in whom this approach is unsuccessful or too slow, *demeclocycline*, a tetracycline derivative which antagonizes the renal tubule effects of ADH, may prove beneficial. Its use will allow liberalization of water intake. The major side effect is photosensitivity; furthermore, its use should be avoided in patients with substantial liver or kidney disease. Other therapeutic maneuvers for SIADH, such as *lithium carbonate* administration (which also interferes with the renal action of ADH) or chronic urea loading (which promotes osmotic diuresis), have been shown to be helpful to some patients.

Other Disorders Associated with Isovolemic Hyponatremia. Patients with *hypothyroidism* may develop hypotonic hyponatremia. The mechanism of the apparent water retention is not fully understood although reduced distal fluid delivery and/or elevated ADH levels have been described in various patients. The latter presumptively reflects the non-osmotic stimulation of ADH release by the reduced cardiac output in myxedema. In addition, excess Na^+ entry into cells and its binding to the increased myxedematous ground substances have been suggested as mechanisms whereby Na^+ may be sequestered. In any case, the hypotonicity is readily corrected with thyroid hormone replacement.

A relatively rare group of patients may have a *"reset osmostat"* and persist with chronic hyponatremia of moderate degree. Such patients are often elderly and poorly nourished, and may have serious underlying diseases. ADH secretion appears to be qualitatively intact though set at a lower threshold of plasma osmolality than normal. Renal function is usually normal (Table 3–4). Thus, such patients dilute and concentrate normally in response to water loads and dehydration, respectively, even though their "normal" serum Na^+ concentration may prefer to remain at the level of 120 to 130 mEq/liter.

More than 20 liters of water a day can be drunk by a normal adult without taxing the kidney's excretory ability.

Occasionally, patients may ingest sufficient free water to noticeably dilute their serum Na^+ concentration. An adult with normal renal function and normal ADH release may drink more than 20 liters of water a day without overwhelming the kidney's ability to excrete this load of solute-free water. Thus, primary polydipsia rarely leads to hypotonic hyponatremia. Generally, another factor contributes to the hypotonicity seen in the severely polydipsic patient. Examples include *psychotic disorders* in which ADH release may be mediated by higher cortical, nonosmotic factors. Other patients may have *diuretic-induced* diluting defects, or *chronic renal insufficiency* with limited delivery of filtrate to the diluting segments. In such instances, increased drinking or free-water infusion usually predisposes to hyponatremia and should be avoided.

REFERENCES

Anatomy of the Body Fluids

Landis, E., and Pappenheimer, J. R.: Exchange of substances through the capillary walls. *In* Hamilton, W. F., and Dow, P., eds.: Handbook of Physiology, Section 2, Vol. 2: Circulation, American Physiological Society, Washington, D.C., 1963.
Classic treatise on the forces governing capillary fluid and solute movements.

Macknight, A. D. C., and Leaf, A.: Regulation of cellular volume. Physiol. Rev. 57:510–573, 1977.
A review of the relationships between cell volume and transcellular ionic gradients.

Maffly, R. H.: The body fluids: Volume, composition, and physical chemistry. *In* Brenner, B. M., and Rector, F. C., Jr., eds.: The Kidney, 2nd Edition. W. B. Saunders Co., Philadelphia, 1981.
A comprehensive review of the factors governing the volume and composition of the various body fluids.

Thirst and ADH Secretion

Aisenbrey, G. A., Handelman, W. A., Arnold, P., Manning, M., and Schrier, R. W.: Vascular effects of arginine vasopressin during fluid deprivation in the rat. J. Clin. Invest. 67:961–968, 1981.
A study suggesting a physiologic pressor role for ADH in dehydrated states.

Andersson, B.: Regulation of water intake. Physiol. Rev. 58:582–603, 1978.
Excellent discussion of the physiological control of drinking.

Robertson, G. L., and Berl, T.: Pathophysiology of water metabolism. *In* Brenner, B. M., and Rector, F. C., Jr., eds.: The Kidney, 3rd Edition. W. B. Saunders Co., Philadelphia, 1986.
An up-to-date discussion of thirst and the neurophysiology of ADH secretion as well as the related clinical disorders.

Hypernatremia

Covey, C. M., and Arieff, A. I.: Disorders of sodium and water metabolism and their effects on the central nervous system. *In* Brenner, B. M., and Stein, J. H., eds.: Contemporary Issues in Nephrology, Vol. 1: Sodium and Water Homeostasis. Churchill Livingstone, Inc., New York, 1978.
Discussion of clinical manifestations and altered CNS composition associated with hyper- and hyponatremia.

Sridhar, C. B., Calvert, G. D., and Ibbertson, H. K.: Syndrome of hypernatremia, hypodipsia, and partial diabetes insipidus: A new interpretation. J. Clin. Endocrinol. Metab. 38:890–901, 1974.
This paper considers the rare patient with hypodipsia in the light of associated renal concentrating defects.

Central and Nephrogenic Diabetes Insipidus

Baylis, P. H., and Heath, D. A.: Water disturbances in patients treated with oral lithium carbonate. Ann. Intern. Med. 88:607–609, 1978.
Clinical study which outlines the range of abnormality in water metabolism associated with lithium carbonate ingestion.

Berl, T., Linas, S. L., Aisenbrey, G. A., and Anderson, R. J.: On the mechanism of polyuria in potassium depletion. J. Clin. Invest. 60:620–625, 1977.
A study incriminating polydipsia in the early stages of the polyuria caused by potassium depletion.

Fine, L. G., Schlondorff, D., Trizna, W., Gilbert, R. M., and Bricker, N. S.: Functional profile of the isolated uremic nephron. J. Clin. Invest. 61:1519–1527, 1978.
Basic study of the pathophysiology of the renal resistance to ADH in uremia.

Hollinshead, W. H.: The interphase of diabetes insipidus. Proc. Mayo Clin. 39:92–100, 1964.
Description of the tri-phasic response of ADH secretion to hypothalamic-pituitary injury.

Leaf, A.: Neurogenic diabetes insipidus. Kidney Int. 15:572–580, 1979.
Excellent review of the syndrome including etiologic factors.

Robertson, G. L., Aycinena, P., and Zerbe, R. L.: Neurogenic disorders of osmoregulation. Am. J. Med. 72:339–353, 1982.
Excellent presentation of information obtained with the plasma radioimmunoassay for ADH.

Singer, I., and Forrest, J. N.: Drug induced states of nephrogenic diabetes insipidus. Kidney Int. 10:82–95, 1976.
Good general review of the pathophysiology of the major pharmacologic causes of nephrogenic diabetes insipidus.

Zusman, R. M., Keiser, H. R., and Handler, J. S.: Vasopressin stimulated prostaglandin E biosynthesis in the toad urinary bladder. J. Clin. Invest. 60:1339–1347, 1977.
Zusman, R. M., Keiser, H. R., and Handler, J. S.: Inhibition of vasopressin-stimulated prostaglandin E biosynthesis by chlorpropamide in the toad urinary bladder. J. Clin. Invest. 60:1348–1353, 1977.
These two articles provide an explanation as to how renal prostaglandins oppose ADH action and how inhibitors of prostaglandin synthesis, including chlorpropamide, may enhance ADH action.

Isotonic and Hypertonic Hyponatremia

Katz, M.: Hyperglycemia-induced hyponatremia—calculation of expected serum sodium depression. N. Engl. J. Med. 289:843–844, 1973.
Short paper describing a means of calculating the fall in serum sodium concentration in hypertonic hyponatremia of diabetes mellitus.

Tarail, R., Buchwald, K. W., Holland, J. F., and Selaw, R. Y.: Misleading reduction of serum sodium and chloride associated with hyperproteinemia in patients with multiple myeloma. Proc. Soc. Exp. Biol. Med. 110:145–148, 1962.
Early description of isotonic hyponatremia with hyperproteinemia.

Hypotonic Hyponatremia Associated with Sodium and Water Loss

Arhraf, N., Locksley, R., and Arieff, A. I.: Thiazide induced hyponatremia associated with death or neurological damage in outpatients. Am. J. Med. 70:1163–1168, 1981.
Discussion of diuretic associated hyponatremia; results suggest that the syndrome may occur with little perceptible volume contraction.

Morgan, D. B., Ball, S. R., Thomas, T. H., and Lee, M. B.: Sodium losing renal disease. Quart. J. Med. 47:21–34, 1978.
Case reports with review of a rare cause of hypotonic hyponatremia.

Fichman, M. P., Vorherr, H., Kleeman, C. R., and Telfer, N.: Diuretic induced hyponatremia. Ann. Intern. Med. 75:853–863, 1971.
Schrier, R. W., and Linas, S. L.: Mechanisms of the defect in water excretion in adrenal insufficiency. Miner. Electrol. Metab. 4:1–7, 1980.
Good review of the pathophysiology of hyponatremia with adrenal disease.

Stein, J. H., Osgood, R. W., Boonjarern, S., Cox, J. W., and Ferris, T. F.: Segmental sodium reabsorption in rats with mild and severe volume depletion. Am. J. Physiol. 227:351–359, 1974.
Basic study demonstrating reduced GFR and enhanced proximal fluid reabsorption in severe volume depletion.

Weitzman, R., Farnsworth, L., McPhee, R., Wang, C. C., and Bennett, C. M.: The effect of opposing osmolar and volume stimuli on plasma arginine vasopressin in man. Miner. Electrol. Metab. 1:43–47, 1978.
Data regarding the competing forces for volume and osmolar homeostasis in volume depletion.

Hypotonic Hyponatremia Associated with Edematous States

Bell, N. H., Schedl, H. P., and Bartter, F. C.: An explanation for abnormal water retention in congestive heart failure. Am. J. Med. 36:351–360, 1964.
A classic study suggesting a role for enhanced proximal reabsorption in the maintenance of hyponatremia in heart failure.

Bichet, D., Szatalowicz, V., Chaimovitz, L., and Schrier, R. W.: Role of vasopressin in abnormal water excretion in cirrhotic patients. Ann. Intern. Med. 96:413–417, 1982.

Szatalowicz, V. L., Arnold, D. E., Chamovitz, C., Bichet, D., Berl, T., and Schrier, R. W.: Radioimmunoassay of plasma arginine vasopressin in hyponatremic patients with congestive heart failure. N. Engl. J. Med. 305:263–266, 1981.
Two papers by this group of investigators which document elevated plasma ADH levels in patients with cirrhosis and heart failure.

Syndrome of Inappropriate ADH Secretion

Bartter, W. C., and Schwartz, W. B.: The syndrome of inappropriate secretion of antidiuretic hormone. Am. J. Med. 42:790–806, 1967.
Original description of this disorder.

Beck, L. H.: Hypouricemia in the syndrome of inappropriate antidiuretic hormone secretion. N. Engl. J. Med. 301:528–530, 1979.
Description of the hypouricemia associated with SIADH.

Forrest, J. N., Jr., Cox, M., Hong, C., Morrison, G., Bia, M., and Singer, I.: Superiority of demeclocycline over lithium in the treatment of chronic syndrome of inappropriate secretion of antidiuretic hormone. N. Engl. J. Med. 298:173–177, 1978.
A comprehensive discussion of the chronic therapy of SIADH.

Hantman, D., Rossier, B., Zohlman, R., and Schrier, R. W.: Rapid correction of hyponatremia in the syndrome of inappropriate secretion of antidiuretic hormone. Ann. Intern. Med. 78:870–875, 1973.
The acute therapy of symptomatic hypotonic hyponatremia with furosemide and hypertonic saline.

Leaf, A., Bartter, F. C., Santos, R. F., and Wrong, O.: Evidence in man that urinary electrolyte loss induced by pitressin is a function of water retention. J. Clin. Invest. 32:868–878, 1953.
Study of pathophysiology of water and sodium excretion with ADH excess.

Martinez-Maldonado, M.: Inappropriate secretion of antidiuretic hormone of unknown origin. Kidney Int. 17:554–567, 1980.
Contemporary review with an emphasis on the systemic diseases underlying SIADH.

Hypotonic Hyponatremic Disorders Associated with Near-Normal Extracellular Volume

Defronzo, R. A., Goldberg, M., and Agus, Z. A.: Normal diluting capacity in hyponatremic patients. Ann. Intern. Med. 84:538–542, 1976.
A description of the reset osmostat.

Skowsky, W. R., and Kikucki, T. A.: The role of vasopressin in the impaired water excretion of myxedema. Am. J. Med. 64:613–621, 1978.
Study of the factors involved in generating and maintaining hyponatremia with myxedema.

4

Regulation and Disorders of Extracellular Fluid Volume

One of the major functions of the kidney is to maintain *extracellular fluid (ECF)* volume relatively constant in spite of large variations in salt and water intake. This regulation is remarkably precise in most people. However, in some patients ECF volume is not maintained within normal limits. When salt retention is mild, hypertension can be present; when salt retention is more marked there will be edema. In other patients, there is a tendency to lose salt; thus blood pressure and ECF volume will be abnormally low.

NORMAL PHYSIOLOGY

As discussed in detail in Chapter 3, the osmolality of body fluids is precisely controlled by the vasopressin system. As a consequence the volume of any compartment will be determined by the total amount of *osmoles* in that compartment. Under normal conditions, thirst and water excretion will be adjusted so as to maintain normal ECF osmolality. An increase in ECF osmoles will lead to increased thirst and renal water retention, which will result in expansion of ECF volume. Conversely, a decrease in ECF osmoles will lead to decreased thirst and enhanced renal water excretion, which will result in contraction of ECF volume. Thus, regulation of ECF volume involves regulation of ECF osmoles. Greater than 90 percent of the osmoles in the ECF space are salts of sodium. Many of these exist in concentrations too small to affect ECF volume, i.e., sodium lactate, sodium citrate, etc. Other sodium salts must maintain their concentration within very narrow limits in order to subserve various homeostatic functions other than ECF volume regulation, i.e., sodium bicarbonate, sodium phosphate. The major salt whose intake and excretion regulates ECF volume is *sodium chloride.*

ECF volume is regulated by the balance between sodium intake and renal excretion of sodium. Figure 4–1 demonstrates normal maintenance of sodium balance. Initially the subject is in balance on a 10 mEq sodium diet as shown by the constant weight and intake equal to excretion. When the diet is changed to 150 mEq sodium (point A), there will be a gradual increase in weight which is totally the result of an increase in ECF volume. This is because the ingested sodium is distributed only in the ECF space and does not enter the intracellular compartment. Only when ECF volume is expanded will renal sodium excretion increase. As long as intake exceeds excretion *(positive balance)*, ECF volume, body weight, and renal sodium excretion will continue to rise (point B). After a few days ECF volume will have risen

Changes in extracellular fluid volume cause changes in renal salt excretion; the mechanisms are multifactorial.

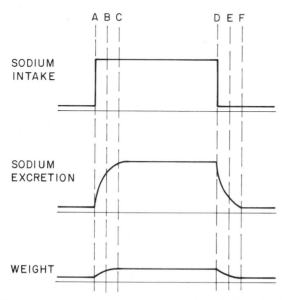

Figure 4–1. Effect of changing sodium intake on body weight and sodium excretion. (Adapted from Reineck, H. J., and Stein, J. H.: Renal regulation of extracellular fluid volume. *In* Brenner, B. M., and Stein, J. H., eds.: Contemporary Issues in Nephrology, Vol. I: Sodium and Water Homeostasis. Churchill Livingstone, Inc., New York, 1978.)

sufficiently such that renal sodium excretion is equal to sodium intake (point C). At this point the person is *in balance* on a 150 mEq sodium diet excreting 150 mEq of sodium per day. This increase in sodium excretion is at the expense of a 1-kg increase in body weight (1-liter increase in ECF volume). When the diet is reduced to 10 mEq sodium (point D), the sequence occurs in reverse. Weight and ECF volume decrease, which leads to a decrease in sodium excretion (point E). After a few days, the person comes into balance with sodium excretion equal to sodium intake and ECF volume remains constant (point F). Thus, major changes in dietary salt intake lead to only small changes in ECF volume because these small changes lead to large changes in salt excretion. The mechanisms by which changes in ECF volume lead to changes in renal salt excretion will now be considered.

Afferent Mechanisms. The regulation of renal salt excretion involves afferent mechanisms that sense the ECF volume and efferent mechanisms that effect the changes in salt handling by the kidney. Although we speak of ECF volume regulation, it is more likely *plasma volume* that is sensed. Under normal conditions, plasma volume will be related to ECF volume. Any salt which is retained will be distributed proportionately between the intravascular and extravascular compartments of the ECF. In certain pathologic states (which are discussed in this chapter) this relationship is altered.

The *low pressure volume receptors* found in the great veins and atria provide a sensitive mechanism for monitoring plasma volume. These veins have a large capacitance and as such are highly distensible. Small changes in central venous pressure can lead to large changes in the size of these vessels, which are then detected by nerve receptors. Evidence for the importance of these receptors in salt excretion comes from the correlation between central venous pressure and sodium excretion. Maneuvers that increase central venous filling, such as weightlessness, recumbency, water immersion, or exposure to cold, all lead to increased salt excretion, whereas maneuvers that decrease central venous filling, such as positive-pressure respirators, assuming the upright position, and leg tourniquets, all lead to sodium retention. Nerve pathways from the great veins and atria lead to the central nervous system, primarily the hypothalamus.

In addition to their neurogenic response, the atria of the heart respond to an increase in blood volume by releasing a small peptide hormone (about 28 amino acids long) called atrial natriuretic peptide (ANP). The atrial myocytes contain many granules (up to 600/cell) that contain the prohormone for ANP. When the atria are distended by an increase in blood volume or pressure, these granules fuse with the plasma membrane and release ANP. ANP has many hemodynamic, renal and endocrine effects. First, ANP induces profound vasodilation and can overcome the effect of any vasoconstrictor that may be present. Second, ANP causes natriuresis and diuresis, in part by its ability to increase the glomerular filtration rate as well as by inhibiting salt transport in the collecting duct. Finally, ANP reduces the circulating concentrations of renin, aldosterone and antidiuretic hormone. Thus, an increased circulating ANP level induces vasodilation and causes natriuresis and diuresis (both directly and by diminishing the major antinatriuretic and antidiuretic hormone concentrations) and thereby tends to restore the circulating blood pressure and volume to normal.

The importance of afferent mechanisms other than the low pressure volume receptors is obvious from a number of situations. The most straightforward of these is the opening and closing of an arteriovenous (AV) fistula. When large AV fistulae are closed acutely, sodium excretion increases accompanied by no change in plasma volume and actually a decrease in central venous filling. Cardiac output, stroke volume, and heart rate all fall, but diastolic blood pressure (BP) rises. Thus, in some way the kidney has responded to a change in the arterial circulation, presumably diastolic BP. When the fistula is reopened, sodium excretion decreases in response to a lowered diastolic BP, in spite of increased central venous filling and cardiac output. A similar discrepancy between central venous filling and renal salt regulation occurs in congestive heart failure. Here central venous filling is increased in the setting of renal salt retention (see below).

These observations have led to the hypothetical concept of an *effective arterial volume*, the fullness of the arterial vascular tree relative to its capacity. It is a balance between the cardiac output and the peripheral resistance. In situations where peripheral vascular resistance remains constant, effective arterial volume will be determined by cardiac output. However, in a number of conditions (AV fistula, peripheral vasodilation) cardiac output increases but the size of the "arterial capacity" increases even more. In this setting effective arterial volume is reduced and the kidneys retain sodium.

The balance between peripheral vascular resistance and cardiac output is called "effective arterial volume."

Baroreceptors present in the aorta and carotid sinus provide a mechanism for sensing effective arterial volume. These receptors perceive changes in effective arterial volume and relay the message to the central nervous system where sympathetic output is altered in such a way as to modify peripheral and renal vascular resistances.

Baroreceptors present in the juxtaglomerular apparatus of the kidney provide an additional mechanism for sensing effective arterial volume. In response to a decreased renal perfusion pressure or β-sympathetic activation, *renin* release by the kidneys is increased. Increased plasma renin leads to increased rates of conversion of *angiotensinogen* to *angiotensin I* which is then converted to *angiotensin II*. Angiotensin II plays a key role in volume homeostasis by multiple mechanisms: (1) renal vasoconstriction; (2) stimulation of *aldosterone* secretion by the adrenal gland; (3) stimulation of sodium transport by the renal tubule; and (4) stimulation of *prostaglandin* production by the kidneys.

In summary, alterations in plasma volume are sensed both on the venous and arterial sides of the circulation. Sensors on the venous side perceive the level of central venous filling via stretch receptors in the great veins and atria. Sensors on the arterial side perceive effective arterial volume which is the filling of the arterial circulation by the cardiac output relative to its capacity. Nerve traffic from the venous and arterial baroreceptors is integrated in the hypothalamus and appropriate efferent pathways are activated. These include alterations in sympathetic nerve activity, which is transmitted to the kidneys through the renal nerves, and the secretion of hormonal factors ("natriuretic hormone") capable of modifying tubule reabsorption of sodium. Stretch of atrial myocytes stimulates the secretion of atrial natriuretic peptide, which accelerates salt excretion by increasing GFR and, possibly, by inhibiting sodium transport in the collecting duct. Activation of the renal baroreceptors affects the secretion of renin, which in turn affects plasma levels of angiotensin II, aldosterone, and prostaglandins. In addition to these neurogenic and hormonal factors, the arterial blood pressure and the physical properties of blood (hematocrit, plasma protein concentrations) may directly enhance the excretion of salt by the kidneys.

Efferent Mechanisms (Fig. 4–2). Exactly how the efferent mechanisms lead to alterations in sodium excretion is a topic that has attracted much investigation. Initially, it was thought that renal salt excretion could be regulated by changes in glomerular filtration rate (GFR). Normally, approximately 25,000 mEq of sodium are filtered per day with daily sodium excretion ranging between 10 and 300 mEq. It was reasoned that small changes in GFR would lead to large changes in sodium excretion if the rate of tubule sodium reabsorption remained constant. This, however, is not the case. When GFR is altered in the absence of changes in ECF volume, the renal tubules regulate sodium reabsorption to match GFR. This phenomenon, known as *glomerulotubular balance*, prevents even large changes in GFR from leading to changes in sodium excretion. It follows therefore that the various

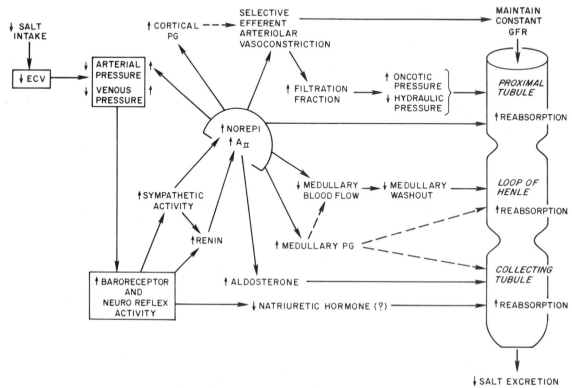

Figure 4–2. Afferent and efferent factors involved in changing renal salt excretion in response to a change in salt intake. Norepi = norepinephrine; AII = angiotensin II; PG = prostaglandins; dashed lines = inhibitory effects of prostaglandins.

efferent mechanisms must in some way affect tubule reabsorption of sodium independently of the GFR.

Proximal Tubule. Expansion of ECF volume depresses, while contraction of ECF volume enhances, reabsorption of NaCl in the proximal tubule. A variety of physical, neurogenic, and hormonal factors mediate these responses of proximal tubule reabsorption to alterations in ECF volume.

One profound and fundamental mechanism regulating proximal reabsorption is the sum of the hydraulic and protein oncotic forces acting across the peritubular capillaries. These forces are responsible for the transfer of the tubule reabsorbate from the renal interstitium into the capillary circulation. Alteration of these forces will change the capillary uptake of reabsorbate and secondarily modify the rate of tubule reabsorption. The overall change in tubule reabsorption is mediated in part by alteration of the permeability of the tight junction connecting the tubule cells, which thus serves to modulate the backleak of some of the transported solutes (see Fig. 1–13), and in part by an effect of peritubular protein concentration on the transcellular transport of NaCl (see Chapter 2). The peritubular hydraulic pressure, which is a function of the arterial blood pressure and renal vascular resistance, is normally 8 to 10 mm Hg. The peritubular protein oncotic pressure, which is a function of the systemic plasma protein concentration and the quantity of protein-free ultrafiltrate removed per unit of plasma flow (filtration fraction), is normally 35 to 40 mm Hg. Thus, the excess of oncotic pressure relative to hydraulic pressure favors capillary uptake of reabsorbate. Selective vasoconstriction of the efferent (postglomerular) arteriole will lower the peritubular hydraulic pressure and, by raising the filtration fraction, will increase the peritubular oncotic pressure. Thus, both capillary uptake and tubule reabsorption will be stimulated. Renal vasodilation has the opposite effect.

Massive volume expansion or volume depletion leads to dilution or concentration of plasma albumin in the systemic vessels and in the renal peritubular capillaries. However, this is probably of importance only in gross alterations of volume status, because minor changes in ECF volume (salt intake) do not lead to detectable changes in plasma protein concentration. These minor changes in salt intake do, however, lead to changes in renal vascular resistance which will secondarily affect peritubular capillary physical factors (Fig. 4–2). Mild volume depletion sensed by both the venous and arterial systemic baroreceptors leads to increased sympathetic tone. Release of *norepinephrine* will cause renal vasoconstriction. *Renin release,* increased by β *adrenergic stimulation* and by *decreased renal perfusion pressure,* leads to increased levels of *angiotensin II.* Increased levels of angiotensin II and norepinephrine result in renal vasoconstriction, usually with the efferent arteriole constricting to a greater extent than the afferent arteriole. This leads to a decrease in renal blood flow (RBF) with maintenance of normal GFR. The increase in filtration fraction (defined as GFR/RBF) will result in a normal amount of protein-free ultrafiltrate being removed from a decreased volume of blood, which leads to a higher concentration of protein in the blood leaving the glomerulus and entering the peritubular capillaries. In addition, the increase in renal vascular resistance lowers the peritubular capillary hydraulic pressure. Both of

The excess of oncotic over hydraulic pressures across the peritubular capillary normally favors net uptake of tubule reabsorbate. When this imbalance is augmented even further (as in high filtration fraction states), tubule reabsorption is enhanced, whereas reabsorption is curtailed when filtration fraction is reduced below normal.

these effects increase the rate of proximal tubule salt and water reabsorption.

Recent evidence has demonstrated that angiotensin II and β-adrenergic agonists can stimulate proximal salt reabsorption in the absence of any hemodynamic alterations. These substances, therefore, exert a direct effect on the proximal tubule epithelium. The direct actions of these agents on proximal reabsorption complement and amplify the changes in reabsorption occurring secondarily to their hemodynamic effects.

In the loop of Henle, volume expansion inhibits salt reabsorption.

Loop of Henle. Micropuncture studies have demonstrated that volume expansion inhibits salt reabsorption in the loop of Henle, and that this effect occurs mostly in the deep nephrons. As discussed in detail in Chapter 2, the loop of Henle consists of the thin descending limb, the thin ascending limb, and the thick ascending limb. Superficial nephrons possess only short descending limbs and no thin ascending limbs. The thin descending limb is impermeable to salts, but is very permeable to water. The thin ascending limb is impermeable to water, but highly permeable to NaCl (see Fig. 2–8). Neither of the thin segments is thought to possess active transport mechanisms. The thick ascending limb of the loop of Henle reabsorbs NaCl actively and is also impermeable to water.

Normally, water is reabsorbed from the thin descending limb in response to the high urea and salt concentrations in the medullary interstitium. This causes a high concentration of NaCl in the fluid presented to the thin ascending limb. The high luminal NaCl concentration provides the driving force for passive NaCl reabsorption in this segment. In conditions where medullary blood flow is increased (volume expansion), the medullary osmotic gradient will be "washed out." The lower interstitial urea and NaCl concentrations will lead to a decreased rate of fluid extraction from the thin descending limb. This will result in a lower concentration of NaCl in the fluid presented to the thin ascending limb and, therefore, to less passive NaCl reabsorption. As thin ascending limbs are present only in deep nephrons, medullary blood flow should affect NaCl reabsorption only in these nephrons. However, if the rate of active NaCl reabsorption in the thick ascending limb is also accelerated by increases in luminal NaCl concentration, there also will be an effect, albeit smaller, of medullary blood flow on NaCl reabsorption in superficial nephrons. During periods of salt restriction and decreased medullary "washout," the reverse of the above will occur (Fig. 4–2).

Under normal conditions, medullary washout produced by increases in medullary blood flow is not sufficient to lead to an increase in NaCl excretion. However, if proximal NaCl reabsorption is inhibited and delivery to the loop of Henle is increased, medullary washout will enhance the magnitude of the natriuresis. This explains why water loads, which lead to medullary washout but do not inhibit proximal NaCl reabsorption, do not lead to a natriuresis. If, however, a water load is given before an infusion of saline, the magnitude of the natriuresis is greater than that seen with saline infusion alone.

Collecting Tubule. Because of its location within the kidney, this nephron segment has been difficult to study. However, a number of mechanisms for an effect of volume expansion on the collecting tubule have been described.

The most well-studied effector is *aldosterone*. As discussed, volume contraction stimulates renin secretion which leads to increased levels of angiotensin II. Angiotensin II then causes an increased rate of aldosterone release from the zona glomerulosa of the adrenal gland. Aldosterone stimulates salt reabsorption in the cortical collecting tubule (Fig. 4–2). This effect is known to require protein synthesis and to involve: (1) an increased amount of enzymes available for ATP synthesis; (2) increased sodium permeability of the luminal membrane; and (3) increases in Na^+-K^+ ATPase on the basolateral membrane (see Fig. 2–12).

Numerous studies have suggested the existence of a natriuretic hormone which may act at the level of the cortical collecting tubule (Fig. 4–2). Atrial peptides, released in response to atrial stretch, have recently been shown to inhibit collecting duct NaCl transport. Studies have also demonstrated that β-adrenergic agonists increase chloride reabsorption in the cortical collecting tubule.

Prostaglandins in Sodium Homeostasis. Prostaglandins and thromboxanes are potent vasoactive compounds and important modulators of renal hemodynamics and kidney salt and water excretion. These unsaturated fatty acid compounds are produced in the kidney from arachidonic acid. The rate-limiting step in prostaglandin synthesis is the release of arachidonic acid from membrane-bound phospholipids under the catalytic action of the enzyme phospholipase A_2 (see Fig. 1–6). This enzyme is under intense physiologic control: it is stimulated by ischemia, calcium, angiotensin II, bradykinin, arginine vasopressin and norepinephrine and is inhibited by potassium, glucocorticoids, and indomethacin. Arachidonic acid is oxidized to two unstable compounds, PGG_2 and PGH_2, under the catalytic action of the enzyme cyclo-oxygenase. Cyclo-oxygenase is the site in prostaglandin synthesis where aspirin, indomethacin, and other nonsteroidal anti-inflammatory agents exert their inhibitory action. PGG_2 and PGH_2 are converted to PGD_2, PGE_2, $PGF_{2\alpha}$, PGI_2, and thromboxane A_2, which are the physiologically active compounds. Overall PGE_2 and $PGF_{2\alpha}$ are the predominant products of endoperoxide metabolism, but the relative concentrations of end products vary from region to region in the kidney. PGE_2 can be converted to $PGF_{2\alpha}$ by action of the enzyme 9-ketoreductase. The activity of this enzyme is stimulated by salt-loading, kinins, and cyclic guanine monophosphate. Thromboxane A_2 is synthesized in relatively small amounts by the kidney, but its synthesis is markedly increased by ureteral or renal venous occlusion and potassium deficiency.

The physiologically active prostaglandins are PGE_2, $PGF_{2\alpha}$, and PGI_2.

When infused into the renal artery prostaglandins are able to inhibit NaCl absorption in the proximal tubule, the loop of Henle, and the collecting tubule. In the proximal tubule the effect is mediated by hemodynamic changes. Prostaglandins (most likely PGI_2) decrease glomerular afferent and efferent arteriolar tone. This leads to increased renal blood flow and decreased filtration fraction which secondarily causes increased hydraulic and decreased oncotic pressures in the peritubular capillaries. As stated earlier, this will inhibit proximal tubule salt and water reabsorption. PGE_2 has also been found to directly inhibit NaCl reabsorption in the thick ascending limb of Henle and in the cortical collecting tubule. Finally, prostaglandins increase medullary blood flow and decrease the osmolality of the medullary interstitium. As stated above, this will decrease water abstraction in the thin descending limb of Henle and secondarily inhibit NaCl reabsorption in the thin ascending limb.

Although all of these actions make prostaglandins ideally suited for mediating the natriuresis of volume expansion, these agents do not function in this fashion, and instead appear to serve more of a counter-regulatory role. In volume-contracted states the production of prostaglandins by the kidney is stimulated by the high levels of angiotensin II and norepinephrine (Figs. 1–7 and 4–2), and is suppressed in volume expansion. Prostaglandins thus counterbalance the vasoconstrictive and sodium-retaining effects of angiotensin II and norepinephrine. If prostaglandin synthesis is inhibited, administrated of angiotensin II leads to marked renal vasoconstriction and sodium retention. Thus, in patients who are volume-expanded or who have normal plasma volume, inhibition of prostaglandin synthesis will have minimal effects on renal vascular resistance and sodium excretion. However, in patients who are actively retaining sodium because of a decreased plasma volume and elevated norepinephrine and angiotensin II levels, inhibition of prostaglandin synthesis can lead to marked renal vasoconstriction, decreased glomerular filtration rate, and salt retention.

Recruitment of Other Homeostatic Mechanisms. It was emphasized above that ECF volume regulation results from regulation of NaCl excretion, while the rates of excretion of other solutes and water are regulated in order to subserve other homeostatic functions. However, when ECF volume is severely compromised the body defends ECF volume at the expense of these other homeostatic functions.

The vasopressin system is an important example of this. Normally ADH secretion and thirst respond in a very sensitive fashion to protect plasma osmolality. In response to decreases in total ECF NaCl content, ADH and thirst will be suppressed, total body water will decrease, and osmolality will return to normal. When, however, total ECF NaCl and volume are severely decreased (sensed by low pressure and high pressure baroreceptors), ADH and thirst will be stimulated by nonosmotic mechanisms (see Chapter 3) so as to protect ECF volume. Thus, marked decreases in ECF volume will be prevented at the expense of decreased plasma osmolality. This sequence of events is an important cause of *hyponatremia*.

Contraction alkalosis results from the kidney's retention of NaHCO₃ to offset ECF volume contraction.

A second example of this phenomenon pertains to acid-base regulation (discussed in detail in Chapter 5). Sodium bicarbonate ($NaHCO_3$) is also an extracellular solute and can function to maintain ECF volume. Under normal circumstances the concentration of $NaHCO_3$ is regulated so as to protect acid-base homeostasis; however, in the presence of marked ECF volume contraction, the kidney will retain $NaHCO_3$. $NaHCO_3$ retention lessens the degree of ECF volume contraction, but leads to a metabolic alkalosis. This condition is referred to as *contraction alkalosis*. Thus, in conditions of marked ECF volume contraction, ECF volume will be defended rather than plasma osmolality or pH.

Figure 4–2 summarizes the homeostatic response to ECF volume contraction. The homeostatic control system would function in the opposite direction in response to ECF volume expansion. This homeostatic system includes many components that interact with each other to ensure that large alterations in dietary salt intake lead to only small changes in ECF volume. Under most conditions this system functions precisely. However, in a number of pathologic conditions, the system fails to protect ECF volume.

EDEMATOUS STATES

The kidney normally responds to increases in sodium intake by increasing sodium excretion, thus preventing more than minor increases in ECF volume. In certain pathologic states, however, this regulatory system breaks down, ingested salt is not excreted by the kidneys, and large increases in ECF volume occur. In some of these conditions the salt retention results from abnormal kidney function, i.e., nephritic syndrome. In other conditions the kidney responds normally to stimuli that are falsely interpreted as contraction of ECF volume, e.g., congestive heart failure. In the case of primary renal salt retention, e.g., nephritic syndrome, ECF volume, total plasma volume, and effective arterial volume are all increased. In the case of secondary salt retention, e.g., congestive heart failure, ECF volume and total plasma volume are increased but the effective arterial volume is reduced. Thus, the distinction between primary renal and secondary salt-retaining states depends on an accurate assessment of the effective arterial volume. Unfortunately, there are no simple measurements, but there are correlating variables such as blood pressure, plasma renin activity, and catecholamine and vasopressin levels. Patients with primary salt retention and increased effective arterial volume will tend to have hypertension, reduced sympathetic activity, and low levels of renin, catecholamines, aldosterone, and vasopressin. In contrast, patients with salt retention secondary to reduced effective arterial volume will tend to have normal or low blood pressure, increased sympathetic nerve activity, and high levels of renin, catecholamines, aldosterone, and vasopressin.

Under normal conditions, 75 percent of ECF is in the *interstitial space* (see Fig. 3–1). Fluid movement between the capillaries and the interstitial space is determined by the balance of the Starling forces between these two compartments:

$$NFP = (P_C - \Pi_C) - (P_I - \Pi_I)$$

where NFP equals the *net filtration pressure,* P the *hydraulic pressure,* Π the *oncotic pressure,* and the subscripts C and I the capillary and interstitial spaces, respectively. The interstitial space has a very low protein oncotic pressure but a subatmospheric hydraulic pressure of -7 mm Hg. This negative hydraulic pressure is maintained by active lymphatic removal of fluid. Capillary hydraulic pressure can be altered by changes in pre- and post-capillary resistances which serve as the homeostatic mechanisms effecting the movement of fluid from the vascular compartment into the interstitial space, or from the interstitial space into the vascular compartment.

The distinction between primary and secondary salt-retaining states is made by an accurate assessment of effective arterial volume.

In certain pathologic states, the amount of interstitial fluid becomes excessive. This condition, *edema*, occurs whenever the mechanisms preventing accumulation of fluid in the interstitium fail. This can be caused by *increased capillary hydraulic pressure, decreased capillary oncotic pressure, or lymphatic disease.*

Congestive Heart Failure (Fig. 4–3). In patients with congestive heart failure (CHF), the kidneys retain NaCl in spite of ECF volume expansion. In this condition, the kidneys are normal, but are retaining salt in response to a message that ECF volume is contracted. The origin of this message has attracted much research.

In most forms of CHF, cardiac output is decreased *(low-output CHF)* while venous filling pressures and volumes are increased. The elevated venous filling pressures are certainly not responsible for salt retention and should lead to a natriuresis in normal patients. However, chronic dilation of the atria, as is present in CHF, decreases their sensitivity to distension and explains why the atrial distension does not lead to natriuresis.

The sodium retention in low-output CHF appears to result from a decreased effective arterial volume. The baroreceptors in the aorta and carotid arteries sense that cardiac output is low. These receptors must sense a pulse contour that reflects effective arterial volume because they clearly cannot merely sense blood pressure; blood pressure is frequently not depressed and in hypertensive patients is

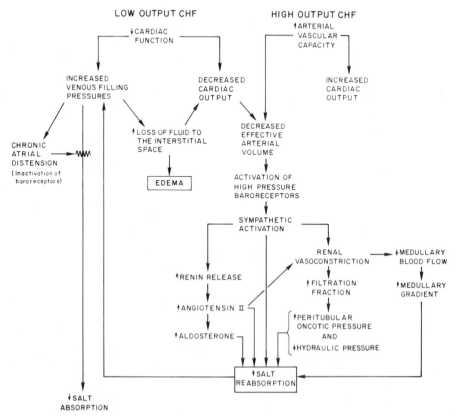

Figure 4–3. Afferent and efferent factors involved in changing renal salt excretion in congestive heart failure (CHF).

elevated. As discussed, effective arterial volume is the balance between the cardiac output and the capacity of the arterial vascular tree. In low-output CHF the decrease in effective arterial volume is caused by decreased cardiac output.

In a number of disorders referred to as *high-output CHF*, salt retention occurs in the presence of a high cardiac output. The primary event in these conditions is an increase in arterial vascular capacity which leads to a decreased peripheral vascular resistance. The heart responds to this decrease in *afterload* with an increase in cardiac output. Because cardiac output does not increase sufficiently to balance the increase in vascular capacity, however, effective arterial volume is decreased and renal salt retention occurs. This leads to increased venous filling pressures and a further increase in cardiac output. In patients with normal hearts, cardiac output eventually increases sufficiently such that effective arterial volume returns to normal. In some patients, however, cardiac output cannot increase to the extent demanded until pathologic levels of venous filling pressure are reached. These patients will be in heart failure (with marked salt retention) with an increased cardiac output. Examples of this condition are *AV fistula, thyrotoxicosis, anemia, beriberi,* and the administration of *peripheral vasodilators.*

The high venous pressures in CHF increase hydraulic pressures in peripheral capillaries and thus lead to an increased rate of interstitial fluid formation. In addition, high venous pressures prevent the return of lymph by inhibiting the emptying of the thoracic duct. Both of these factors tend to increase interstitial volume at the expense of effective arterial volume and thus enhance renal salt retention.

In response to decreased effective arterial volume, nerve impulses originating in the arterial baroreceptors are relayed to the medulla oblongata and hypothalamus, which then increase sympathetic nerve outflow. This leads to renal vasoconstriction, an increase in filtration fraction with associated changes in peritubular capillary physical forces, decreased medullary blood flow, and increased tubule salt and water reabsorption. The sympathetic activation also leads to renin release with secondary increases in angiotensin II and aldosterone. The roles of natriuretic factors in CHF have not been defined. ADH is elevated in many patients with CHF and can frequently lead to hyponatremia.

Salt retention in CHF leads to further increases in venous filling pressures, which promote an increase in cardiac output (and an increase in effective arterial volume). If untreated, patients with CHF will eventually come into balance. At this point, cardiac output is sufficient for arterial vascular capacity and effective arterial volume is normal, but at the expense of increased venous pressures. As cardiac function decompensates further, the required venous pressures necessary for maintenance of effective arterial volume may lead to peripheral or pulmonary congestion and edema.

Numerous treatment modalities have been developed for patients with CHF (Fig. 4–4). The physician may treat with *positive inotropic agents* such as the *cardiac glycosides,* which will lower venous pressures while cardiac output and effective arterial volume are improved. This will lead to natriuresis. A second treatment approach is the use of *diuretics.* These will also lower venous pressure, but will lower cardiac

Low-output congestive heart failure shows a decreased cardiac output with increased venous filling pressures and volumes. High-output congestive heart failure shows an increased cardiac output with decreased arterial volume and renal salt retention.

Diuretics cause natriuresis despite decreased effective arterial volume by directly inhibiting tubule NaCl reabsorption.

	Venous filling pressures	Cardiac output	Effective arterial volume	NaCl excretion
Cardiac glycosides	↓	↑	↑	↑
Diuretics	↓	↓	↓	↑
Peripheral vasodilators	↓	↑	↓	↓

Figure 4–4. Hemodynamic effects of treatment for congestive heart failure.

output and effective arterial volume as well. Diuretics lead to natriuresis in spite of the decreased effective arterial volume by directly inhibiting tubule NaCl reabsorption. A third treatment choice is an *arterial vasodilator*, which decreases peripheral resistance and thus increases cardiac output. With these agents, venous pressure will decline and cardiac output will increase, but effective arterial volume will decrease. This explains the frequent observation that patients treated with vasodilators have improved hemodynamics (increased cardiac output with decreased venous filling pressures) but retain large amounts of NaCl and become edematous.

In summary, CHF is associated with a decreased effective arterial volume which leads to salt retention. Chronically elevated atrial pressures decrease the sensitivity of the low pressure volume receptors and thus prevent these high atrial pressures from inducing a natriuresis. The elevated venous pressure causes fluid to leave the vascular space and further contribute to the decreased effective arterial volume. These factors lead to renal salt retention all along the nephron. CHF provides an excellent example of an edematous state where the kidney is normal and responds to a decreased effective arterial volume by retaining salt.

Nephritic Syndrome (Fig. 4–5). *Nephritis* is an example of an edematous state in which NaCl retention is caused by an abnormal kidney. The most classic example of this syndrome is acute poststreptococcal glomerulonephritis, with its mild decrease in GFR but intense renal NaCl retention. Therapeutic intervention is frequently required because of complications related to this salt retention (hypertension, pulmonary edema, etc.).

Venous pressures and effective arterial volume are both elevated in nephritis. These should lead to a natriuresis but do not. Serum albumin tends to be decreased from dilution. In addition, GFR is decreased while renal blood flow is normal, which means that filtration fraction is decreased. The combination of a decreased serum albumin and a decreased filtration fraction will lead to decreased peritubular capillary oncotic pressure and should inhibit proximal tubule salt reabsorption. Indeed, studies in experimental models have confirmed that salt reabsorption is inhibited in the proximal tubule and that the site of avid salt retention is in the distal nephron. The mechanism of the distal nephron salt retention in these glomerular diseases is unclear. The renin-angiotensin-aldosterone system is appropriately suppressed in response to the expanded ECF volume.

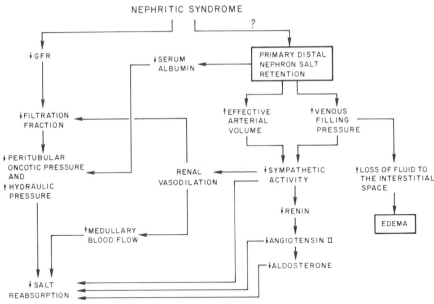

Figure 4–5. Afferent and efferent factors involved in changing renal salt excretion in the nephritic syndrome.

In summary, patients with the nephritic syndrome retain sodium avidly for unclear reasons. Low pressure and high pressure receptors appropriately sense the expanded volume, peritubular capillary physical forces change in such a way as to suppress proximal reabsorption, and the renin-angiotensin-aldosterone system is suppressed. In spite of all these factors, renal salt retention is avid and leads to increased peripheral capillary hydraulic pressure and edema.

Nephrotic Syndrome (Fig. 4–6). The *nephrotic syndrome* is defined clinically as the combination of proteinuria greater than 3.5 gm/day and hypoalbuminemia. This syndrome is also frequently associated with hypercholesterolemia, lipiduria, and edema. The mechanism of this edema has traditionally been ascribed to hypoalbuminemia, but recent studies have suggested a more complicated mechanism.

Hypoalbuminemia deceases the plasma oncotic pressure in peripheral capillaries, and leads to increased loss of fluid from the vascular space into the interstitial space. This is the primary event in classic nephrotic syndrome, and results in a decreased plasma volume. Low-pressure receptors sense decreased venous pressure, while high-pressure receptors sense decreased effective arterial volume. The result is the recruitment of all of the efferent mechanisms discussed earlier in this chapter. Peritubular capillary physical factors are an exception to this, however. In spite of the increased filtration fraction, peripheral hypoalbuminemia results in a decrease in peritubular capillary oncotic pressure, and proximal tubule salt reabsorption is inhibited. Thus, similar to the nephritic syndrome, sodium retention in the nephrotic syndrome results primarily from increased distal tubule reabsorption.

According to the above schema, renal salt retention is caused by a hypoalbuminemia-induced decrease in plasma volume. There are, however, a number of problems with this thesis. One might predict,

In the nephrotic syndrome, edema is due to loss of fluid from vascular into interstitial spaces secondary to massive albuminuria and hypoalbuminemia.

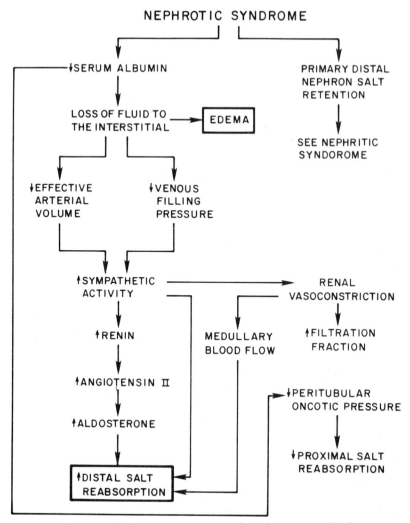

Figure 4–6. Afferent and efferent factors involved in changing renal salt excretion in the nephrotic syndrome.

then, that there would be a good correlation between the level of hypoalbuminemia and the degree of edema. This has never been found to be true. There is a condition known as analbuminemia in which, because of a hepatic synthetic defect, serum albumin is absent in the plasma. Despite the very low plasma oncotic pressure, these patients, who have normal kidneys, are free of edema. The above schema also predicts that measures of plasma volume should be decreased. This has been found to be true in some patients with the nephrotic syndrome who have normal blood pressures, decreased plasma volumes, and high renin and aldosterone levels. However, many patients with the nephrotic syndrome are hypertensive and have increased plasma volumes and low renin and aldosterone levels. In this second group of patients, the pathophysiology of renal salt retention appears to be more similar to that in the nephritic syndrome.

It appears that patients with the nephrotic syndrome possess two mechanisms of salt retention. In one, albuminuria leads to hypoalbuminemia which leads to sequestration of fluid into the interstitial space and a decreased plasma volume. In the other, primary renal salt retention similar to that which occurs in the nephritic syndrome leads to an expanded plasma volume which also leads to sequestration of fluid in the interstitial space (increased peripheral capillary hydraulic pressure). Some patients are dominated by the first mechanism and will have normal blood pressures, decreased plasma volumes, and high renin and aldosterone levels. Other patients are dominated by the second mechanism and will have hypertension, increased plasma volumes, and low renin and aldosterone levels. The presence of two mechanisms of edema formation explains the poor correlation between serum albumin and the magnitude of the edema. It may also explain why patients with analbuminemia who have no primary salt retention are not edematous.

In summary, salt retention and edema formation in the nephrotic syndrome can be the consequence of two independent mechanisms. The first is hypoalbuminemia secondary to albuminuria, which leads to loss of fluid from the vascular space and a decreased plasma volume. The second mechanism is primary renal salt retention secondary to the glomerular injury, similar to that which occurs in the nephritic syndrome.

Cirrhosis (Fig. 4–7). *Cirrhosis* is another example of a disorder in which a normal kidney receives an aberrant message of decreased ECF volume and retains salt. Here, however, the afferent mechanisms

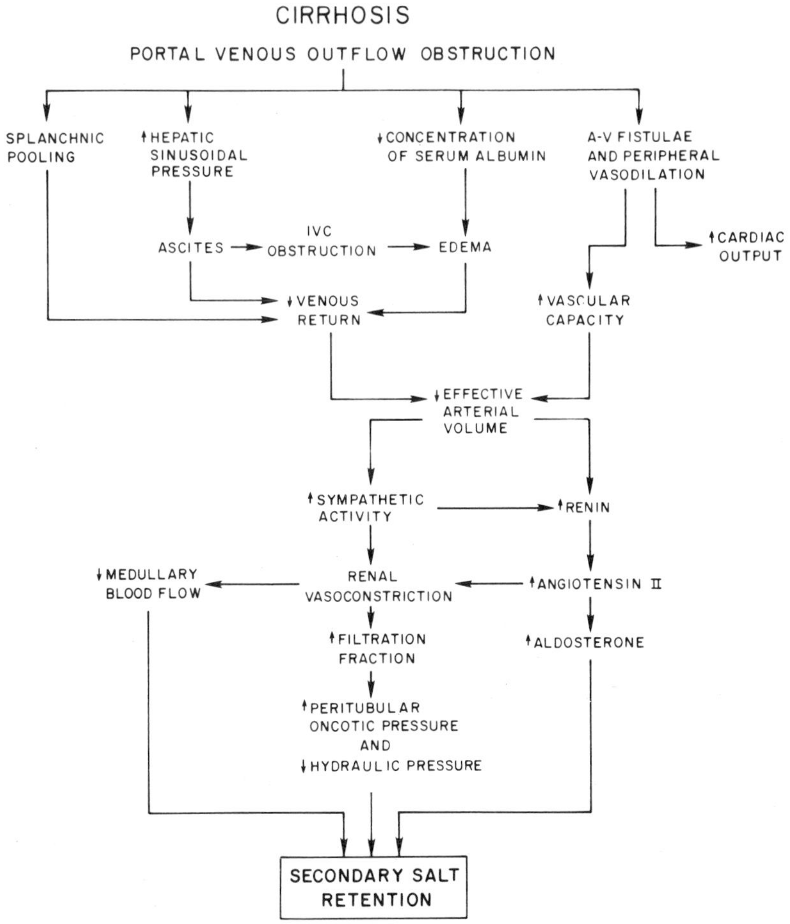

Nephrotic syndrome patients have two mechanisms of salt retention (and edema formation), resulting in differing (and seemingly opposite) symptoms of the disorder.

Figure 4–7. Afferent and efferent factors involved in changing renal salt excretion in cirrhosis of the liver.

involved are extremely complex. The critical event in the development of salt retention, edema, and ascites is obstruction to portal venous outflow. Presinusoidal hepatic diseases such as schistosomiasis and portal vein obstruction do not lead to marked salt retention unless they are associated with postsinusoidal cirrhosis. *Postsinusoidal* hepatic diseases such as *Laennec's cirrhosis* and the *Budd-Chiari syndrome* (hepatic vein occlusion) are associated with marked degrees of salt retention, anasarca, and ascites.

Cirrhosis can in many ways be considered an example of high-output heart failure. For unclear reasons, patients with cirrhosis have a low systemic vascular resistance caused by AV fistulae and peripheral vasodilation. The fistulae are present in skin, muscle, lungs, and the splanchnic circulation. As a consequence cardiac output is shunted through these low resistance vessels. In order for effective arterial volume to be maintained, cardiac output must increase proportionately. Although cirrhotic patients with salt retention do have high cardiac output, it is not high enough to compensate for the increased vascular capacity. A major reason for this inadequate rise in cardiac output is that venous filling pressures cannot increase to the extent required.

There are multiple reasons for inappropriately low venous filling pressures. First, hepatic venous outflow obstruction leads to increased pressures in the hepatic sinusoids, which leads to an increased rate of interstitial fluid formation. When this rate becomes greater than the rate at which lymphatics can return fluid to the vascular space, ascites forms and intravascular volume is depleted. Second, portal venous outflow obstruction leads to sequestration of a large volume of plasma within the splanchnic vessels, which decreases the extrasplanchnic vascular volume. Third, hypoalbuminemia from parenchymal hepatic failure leads to further sequestration of fluid in the interstitial spaces. Fourth, tense ascites can compress the inferior vena cava, resulting in edema formation in the lower extremities. All four of the above factors contribute to decreased filling pressures and thus prevent cardiac output from increasing sufficiently to maintain effective arterial volume. Sodium retained by the kidney does not lead to increased venous filling pressures and increased cardiac output, but rather to ascites and edema formation. There is also some evidence suggesting that intrinsic cardiac function may be decreased in patients with cirrhosis. This would also prevent cardiac output from increasing sufficiently to return effective arterial volume to normal.

"Classic" vs. "overflow" theories of ascites formation in cirrhosis.

According to the above formulation, known as the *classic theory of ascites formation*, salt retention in patients with cirrhosis is caused by decreased effective arterial volume. Some investigators, however, have postulated that effective arterial volume is elevated and that the salt retention is a primary renal event. According to this theory, referred to as the "overflow" hypothesis, hepatic venous outflow obstruction somehow leads to primary renal salt retention which then leads to edema and ascites formation.

The best evidence in favor of primary renal sodium retention is from dog studies where cirrhosis has been induced by chronic feeding of dimethylnitrosamine. In this model it has been shown that salt retention begins before any ascites formation, hypoalbuminemia, change in cardiac output, or change in renin and aldosterone level. In addition, extrasplanchnic blood volume is not decreased. In these dog studies, however, blood pressure tended to decrease and it is not clear that there was not a small decrease in peripheral resistance. This could lead to a decreased effective arterial volume and sodium retention.

The distinction between these two theories in human cirrhotic patients rests on the magnitude of the effective arterial volume. The classic theory predicts that effective arterial volume is decreased, while the overflow theory predicts that effective arterial volume is increased. Although there is not a simple method for measuring effective arterial volume, there are variables which correlate with this parameter and thus allow an educated guess.

Before addressing this question, it is important to emphasize that not all patients with cirrhosis retain sodium; many do not have ascites and are referred to as "compensated." Patients with ascites are referred to as "decompensated" and can be divided into three groups. One group mobilizes ascites (sodium excretion exceeds sodium intake), one group is in sodium balance, and one group actively accumulates ascites (sodium intake exceeds sodium excretion). In examining the mechanism of renal sodium retention in cirrhotic patients, it is important to consider only this last group of patients, because they are the only ones who pathologically retain sodium.

As discussed earlier, renin, aldosterone, ADH, and norepinephrine levels are all elevated in patients with decreased effective arterial volumes and depressed in patients with increased effective arterial volumes. When measured in patients with cirrhosis, these hormone levels are variable. When only patients who are actively retaining sodium are considered, however, renin, aldosterone, ADH, and norepinephrine are elevated. These results suggest that renal salt retention occurs in response to a decreased effective arterial volume.

In addition, patients with cirrhosis and ascites tend to have low-normal blood pressures in spite of high angiotensin II levels. The combination of low-normal blood pressures with marked vasoconstriction further suggests decreased effective arterial volume.

The salt retention in cirrhosis occurs in both the proximal and distal nephrons. Proximal tubule salt retention occurs in spite of a decreased serum albumin. This leads to marked decreases in distal delivery which are associated with defects in free-water clearance and, in some patients, a distal renal tubular acidosis. In spite of all of the defects in ECF volume regulation described above, patients with cirrhosis do regulate their ECF volume, albeit at a different set point. When these patients are immersed in water up to their necks, a large volume of fluid is returned to the central venous system (similar to a large infusion). The patients respond to this procedure with a natriuresis, improvement in free-water clearance, and suppression of renin and aldosterone levels.

Patients with cirrhosis are able to regulate their ECF volume despite the alterations in body fluid homeostasis associated with the disorder.

In summary, patients with cirrhosis are in a state of marked sodium retention. The degree of portal venous outflow obstruction appears to correlate best with the degree of salt retention. Renal salt retention occurs in response to a decreased effective arterial volume. The decreased effective arterial volume results from: (1) sequestration of fluid in the peritoneal cavity (ascites) and splanchnic vessels, and (2) peripheral vasodilation and arteriovenous fistula formation.

ECF VOLUME DEPLETION (TABLE 4–1)

Decreases in salt intake normally lead to only minor decreases in ECF volume because salt excretion falls appropriately. Under certain pathologic conditions, however, marked decreases in ECF volume occur when salt losses exceed salt intake. These conditions can be classified as extrarenal or renal, based on the site of salt loss (Table 4–1). *Extrarenal* causes usually involve loss of NaCl through the *gastrointestinal tract*, but can also involve loss through the *skin*. In addition, intravascular volume depletion can occur when NaCl is sequestered from the vascular compartment into a *"third space,"* such as the peritoneum, skin, or injured muscle. In all these conditions, a normal kidney responds to the marked volume contraction by increasing sodium reabsorption. This can be detected clinically by a low urinary sodium concentration (<10 mEq/liter) or a low fractional excretion of sodium $<.01$ ($\frac{U_{Na}\ P_{CR}}{U_{CR}\ P_{Na}}$). An exception to this rule is during active vomiting. The loss of HCl generates excess bicarbonate in plasma, which is partially excreted into the urine as $NaHCO_3$. Thus, the urine has a high urine sodium concentration and fractional sodium excretion, despite a contracted ECF volume and otherwise normal kidneys. This same phenomenon can be seen when other nonreabsorbable anions, e.g., carbenicillin or salicylate, promote an obligatory loss of cation (Na^+, K^+, NH_4^+) into the urine. In these circumstances a low urine Cl^- concentration (<10 mEq/liter) provides the best index of ECF volume contraction. These urinary indices demonstrate that the kidney is functioning normally and that the ECF volume depletion must have an extrarenal cause.

Renal causes of volume depletion are associated with inappropriately elevated urinary Na^+ and Cl^- concentrations (>20 mEq/liter) and fractional excretion of sodium (>.01). Renal causes of volume depletion can be classified as intrinsic and extrinsic processes.

Table 4–1. CAUSES OF EXTRACELLULAR FLUID VOLUME DEPLETION

Extrarenal
    GI loss—vomiting, diarrhea, fistula drainage, laxatives
    Skin loss
    Sequestration
        Peritonitis, injured skin or muscle

Renal
    Intrinsic
        Chronic renal disease
        Medullary cystic disease
        Interstitial nephritis
        Postobstructive uropathy
        Analgesic nephropathy
        Diuretic phase of acute tubular necrosis
        Proximal and distal renal tubular acidosis

    Extrinsic
        Mineralocorticoid deficiency
        Osmotic diuresis (e.g., glycosuria)
        Diuretics

Intrinsic renal processes are states in which the kidney is unable to respond to ECF volume contraction because of intrinsic renal disease. The condition most frequently associated with renal salt wasting is *chronic renal failure.* Patients with chronic renal disease have difficulty conserving salt in the face of dietary restriction because of the continual osmotic diuresis arising from the excretion of nitrogenous waste products through a reduced number of nephrons. The other forms of renal disease in which the kidneys are unusually predisposed toward salt wasting all involve the renal tubules and include: *medullary cystic disease, interstitial nephritis, postobstructive uropathy, analgesic nephropathy,* the *diuretic phase of acute tubular necrosis,* and *proximal and distal renal tubular acidosis.*

Renal causes of volume depletion are classified as intrinsic (e.g., chronic renal failure) or extrinsic (e.g., mineralocorticoid deficiency).

It is important to emphasize that salt wasting is unusual in postobstructive uropathy and the diuretic phase of ATN. Although there are well documented cases of salt wasting in these conditions, the natriuresis can usually be explained by salt retention during the period of renal failure and the urea osmotic diuresis that ensues upon improvement of renal function. Many times, physicians who think a patient is diuresing too quickly will infuse large volumes of saline into these already volume-expanded patients, leading to further volume expansion and increasing diuresis. The diuresis will not stop until the infusion is slowed or stopped.

Causes of renal salt wasting can also be *extrinsic* to the kidney; the renal tubules function normally, but respond to conditions that prevent them from retaining salt. *Mineralocorticoid deficiency* is an important extrinsic cause of salt wasting: the renal tubules function normally but respond to decreased aldosterone by increasing salt excretion. Mineralocorticoid deficiency can be caused by Addison's disease, adrenal biosynthetic defects, or abnormal renal renin production. In some patients aldosterone levels are normal but the distal nephron is unresponsive to aldosterone. Invariably, when salt wastage is secondary to aldosterone deficiency or resistance there will be impaired potassium secretion and hyperkalemia.

Osmotic diuresis will also prevent the kidneys from retaining salt appropriately. This can be caused by retained urea in patients who are recovering from a renal insult, glucose in diabetics, mannitol, or radiocontrast agents. *Diuretic* administration will also lead to inappropriate salt excretion.

The clinical consequences of ECF depletion depend on the magnitude of the salt deficit, the source and acid-base composition of the fluid lost from the body, and the associated physiologic compensatory responses (Table 4–2). Most of the clinical signs and symptoms relate to underfilling of the circulation and reduced cardiac output. The blood pressure may range from low normal to profound shock; there will be an associated tachycardia. Assuming an upright posture will worsen the hypotension and tachycardia, and may induce dizziness or syncope. Central venous pressure, which is a useful index of vascular filling, will be low or zero. Glomerular filtration rate may be reduced, resulting in elevated blood urea nitrogen and creatinine levels. Elevated hematocrit and plasma protein concentration are useful as indices of the extent of volume contraction.

Most of the clinical signs and symptoms of ECF depletion relate to circulatory underfilling and reduced cardiac output.

Table 4–2. CONSEQUENCES OF EXTRACELLULAR FLUID VOLUME DEPLETION

Hemodynamic instability
  Hypotension, tachycardia
  Postural dizziness or syncope
  Decreased central venous pressure
  Decreased glomerular filtration rate
    Increased blood urea nitrogen and creatinine

Hyponatremia
  Increased thirst
  Impaired renal water excretion
    Nonosmotic stimulation of vasopressin secretion
    Decreased salt and water delivery to distal nephron

Potassium disorders
  Hypokalemia
    Increased renin and aldosterone secretion
    Excretion of poorly reabsorbed anions, e.g., bicarbonate,
      carbenicillin, salicylate
  Hyperkalemia
    Low aldosterone secretion
    Aldosterone resistance

Acid-base disorders
  Metabolic alkalosis
    Vomiting, diuretics
  Hyperchloremic acidosis
    Diarrhea, renal disease
  Anion-gap acidosis
    Lactic acidosis secondary to shock

There may also be associated disturbances in the composition of plasma, with dilutional hyponatremia as one of the more frequent. Contraction of ECF volume stimulates thirst and impairs water excretion because of nonosmotic stimulation of vasopressin and decreased delivery of salt and water to the distal diluting segments of the nephron (secondary to decreased GFR and increased fractional reabsorption in the proximal nephron).

ECF volume depletion may also be associated with acid-base disturbances. If the salt and water loss is secondary to vomiting or diuretics there is usually a metabolic alkalosis. If the salt and water loss is secondary to either diarrhea or renal disease (chronic renal insufficiency, renal tubular acidosis) there is frequently a hyperchloremic metabolic acidosis. If the ECF depletion is profound, with shock and tissue ischemia, there may be an anion-gap type of metabolic acidosis due to lactic acid. Finally, there may be disturbances in potassium homeostasis. ECF volume depletion normally results in hyperreninemia and secondary hyperaldosteronism. If the renal tubule is responsive to aldosterone, and sodium salts of poorly reabsorbable anions (bicarbonate, carbenicillin, salicylate) are being excreted, renal potassium wastage and hypokalemia will supervene. Conversely, if there is defective secretion of renin or aldosterone, or if the tubule is resistant to aldosterone, hyperkalemia will occur.

HYPERTENSION

Arterial blood pressure is determined by the cardiac output and peripheral vascular resistance. The cardiac output is controlled by blood volume, venous tone, and myocardial contractility, while peripheral vascular resistance is a complex function of autoregulation of intrinsic vascular tone, the autonomic nervous system, and the action of vasoconstrictors and vasodepressors produced in vessel walls or circulating in plasma.

Control of Blood Pressure. The kidneys participate in the control of blood pressure in several ways. First and most important, by precisely maintaining salt balance the kidneys regulate plasma volume, the filling pressures of the heart, and cardiac output. If the kidneys fail to conserve salt, then ECF volume, plasma volume, cardiac output, and blood pressure will all be reduced. If, on the other hand, the kidneys have difficulty in excreting the dietary salt loads, either because of an intrinsic abnormality of the kidney or because of extrarenal factors (e.g., excess mineralocorticoid hormone), ECF and plasma volumes as well as blood pressure will be increased. Second, the kidney produces several potent vasoactive substances which are capable of profoundly altering vascular resistance. The most important of these is the renin-angiotensin system. During periods of ECF or plasma volume contraction, the combined effects of activation of the renal baroreceptors and increased sympathetic nerve activity result in renin secretion by the kidney and, subsequently, increased circulating levels of angiotensin II. The high levels of angiotensin II increase peripheral vascular resistance and thus help maintain blood pressure in the face of volume contraction and low cardiac output. Inhibition of either the formation or action of angiotensin II under these conditions results in a marked fall in blood pressure. In certain pathologic states usually involving renal ischemia or hypoperfusion, excessive amounts of renin and angiotensin II are produced, resulting in chronic hypertension. Inhibition of the formation or action of angiotensin II will completely correct this form of hypertension.

Blood pressure is reduced if the kidneys fail to conserve salt. Blood pressure is increased if the kidneys fail to excrete salt.

Potent vasoactive prostaglandins, thromboxanes, and kinins are produced within the kidney. These substances clearly play very important roles in regulation of intrarenal vascular resistance, but there is no convincing evidence that they enter the systemic circulation or influence peripheral vascular resistance. There are cells within the renal medulla which contain a potent vasodepressor-neutral lipid. Extracts of the medulla or implants of the medullary cells into the peritoneal cavity will reverse renovascular or salt-overload hypertension in experimental animals. However, the role that this renal medullary factor plays in the normal physiologic control of blood pressure or in the pathogenesis of hypertension is not known. Finally, there are mechano- and chemoreceptors within the kidney that can be activated by changes in stretch, oxygen tension, or ionic composition, and can modify systemic sympathetic nerve activity and peripheral vascular resistance by means of renal afferent nerve pathways to the central nervous system.

Epidemiology. In modern urban or industrial societies blood pressure increases progressively with age and is higher in obese than nonobese individuals. In more rural or primitive societies the progressive rise in blood pressure with age is not seen. In urban societies, hypertension, defined as a diastolic blood pressure greater than 90 mm Hg, affects 15 to 20 percent of the population, while in rural societies the incidence is much lower. Although there are many environmental and societal factors that might contribute to this difference in the incidence of hypertension, differences in dietary salt intake have received much emphasis. Within a given population, however, there is a strong correlation between blood pressure and age and degree of obesity, but no correlation with salt intake. This does not exclude the possibility, however, that certain individuals within a population group have difficulty handling dietary salt loads and, as a consequence, develop salt-dependent hypertension. In the United States the incidence of hypertension increases with age, reaching approximately 20 percent by the age of 50 years. At every age the incidence in blacks is almost twice that in whites.

In the U.S., the incidence of hypertension among blacks is nearly twice that of whites, in all age groups.

Chronic diastolic hypertension (diastolic BP greater than 90 mm Hg) can be either primary or secondary. Primary or essential hypertension has no known cause, tends to cluster in families, has its highest incidence in societies with high dietary salt intake, and accounts for approximately 90 percent of all hypertensive patients. Secondary forms of hypertension have an identifiable cause for the hypertension and account for the remaining 10 percent of hypertensive patients. Chronic renal parenchymal disease accounts for 4 to 5 percent of all hypertension, while renovascular disease accounts for 3 to 4 percent, coarctation of the aorta for 1 percent, primary aldosteronism for 0.5 percent, Cushing's syndrome for 0.2 percent, and pheochromocytoma for 0.2 percent. All other causes of hypertension such as estrogen therapy, hypercalcemia, carcinoid syndrome, lead intoxication, etc., account for less than 1 percent of hypertensive individuals.

Pathophysiology (Table 4–3). Hypertension can be divided into those forms caused primarily by salt retention and overexpansion of ECF and plasma volumes, and those primarily caused by vasoconstriction. Although this simple classification provides a helpful intellectual framework, certain forms of hypertension have both components and do not fit comfortably into such a formulation.

In the salt- or volume-dependent forms of hypertension there is a positive correlation between blood pressure and plasma volume, and as an expression of the volume-expanded state the plasma renin activity is suppressed. Aldosterone secretion may be either high or low, depending on the underlying disease. In primary diseases of the adrenal gland (primary hyperaldosteronism, Cushing's disease), the secretion of mineralocorticoid hormone will be high, and in addition to being volume-expanded and hypertensive, the patient will waste potassium and develop hypokalemic metabolic alkalosis. In acute glomerulonephritis, in patients with tubulointerstitial disease of the kidneys, and in a rare disorder in which NaCl transport in the distal tubule is selectively accelerated, there is hyporeninemic hypoaldosteronism with hyperkalemia and mild hyperchloremic acidosis in association with the hypertension.

Table 4–3. ETIOLOGIC AND PATHOPHYSIOLOGIC FACTORS IN HYPERTENSION

	Plasma Volume	Plasma Renin Activity	Urinary Aldosterone Excretion	Serum K^+
I Primary Volume Overexpansion				
Extrarenal (mineralocorticoid excess)				
Primary hyperaldosteronism	↑	↓	↑	↓
Cushing's syndrome	↑	↓	nl or ↑	↓
Exogenous	↑	↓	↓	↓
Renal				
Acute glomerulonephritis	↑	↓	↓	
Tubulointerstitial nephropathy	↑	↓	↓	↑
Accelerated distal NaCl reabsorption	↑	↓	↓	↑
Liddle's syndrome	↑	↓	↓	↓
II Primary Vasoconstriction				
Pheochromocytoma	↓	↑	nl or ↑	nl
Renovascular				
Renal artery stenosis	↓ or ↑	↑	↑	nl or ↓
Vasculitis	↓	↑	↑	nl or ↓
Coarctation of the aorta	↑	↑	—	—
Estrogens	?	↑	—	—
Preeclampsia	↓	↓	↓	—
Hypercalcemia	?	?	?	—
III Mixed				
Chronic renal insufficiency	↑	var	nl	nl
Essential hypertension				
Low renin	nl	↓	nl	nl
Normal renin	sl ↓	nl	nl	nl
High renin	↓	↑	nl	nl

nl, normal; sl ↓, slightly reduced; ↑, increased; ↓, decreased; var, variable.

    In these primary volume-dependent forms of hypertension, cardiac output is normal and increased peripheral vascular resistance accounts for the elevated blood pressure. The cause of this increased vascular resistance has been ascribed to the phenomenon termed "whole-body autoregulation." According to this view, salt retention and volume expansion tend to increase cardiac output and tissue blood flow. In response, the vascular bed of each organ or tissue tends to autoregulate its resistance upward in order to return blood flow back to a normal level commensurate with the metabolic needs of the tissue. An alternative view is that in response to volume expansion and activation of the baroreceptors, an inhibitor of the Na^+-K^+ ATPase pump is released from the hypothalamus into the circulation. This circulating Na^+ transport inhibitor acts on the renal tubule and restores salt balance. However, the inhibitor also acts on nonrenal tissues such as vascular smooth muscle and causes a rise in intracellular Na^+ and a fall in the cell membrane electrical potential difference. The extrusion of Ca^{++} from the cell, which is directly coupled to Na^+ entry and is driven by the electrochemical gradient for Na^+, will be reduced; as a consequence, intracellular Ca^{++} will rise. This causes increased vascular

Two views of "whole-body autoregulation" of vascular resistance.

tone and reactivity and elevated blood pressure. In support of the view that a circulating Na^+ transport inhibitor could participate in elevation of the blood pressure is the observation that infusions of digoxin (a potent inhibitor of Na^+-K^+ ATPase) increase peripheral vascular resistance and raise blood pressure. An inhibitor of the Na^+-K^+ ATPase enzyme system has been found in plasma by several investigators, although not by all. Thus its existence is still controversial. Studies by investigators who have been able to measure circulating levels of the inhibitor have shown the levels to increase with salt loads, to decrease with salt restriction, and to be high in many patients with hypertension. Since the secretion of this inhibitor is presumed to be triggered by increased pressure or stretch in the atrial and arterial baroreceptors, it is not clear whether the increased levels of the inhibitor cause the hypertension or whether they are simply a passive consequence of the elevated venous and arterial blood pressures.

Is there a Na^+-K^+ ATPase pump inhibitor?

In contrast to the above forms of hypertension which are secondary to salt retention and volume expansion are other forms which are caused by *primary vasoconstriction*. A classic example of this form of hypertension is that caused by pheochromocytoma with increased secretion of norepinephrine. This potent vasoconstrictor increases peripheral vascular resistance and elevates blood pressure. Although the cause of this form of hypertension is extrarenal, the kidneys do participate in a complex way. As the blood pressure rises the kidneys respond by increasing salt excretion in order to reduce plasma volume and restore blood pressure to normal. Plasma volume is in fact always reduced in hypertensive patients with pheochromocytoma. This compensatory response on the part of the kidneys, however, is incomplete and the blood pressure remains high. The reason for the incomplete renal response is the fact that high levels of catecholamines cause renal vasoconstriction and directly stimulate tubule reabsorption of salt. In addition, the renal vasoconstriction stimulates the secretion of renin and the formation of angiotensin II. Thus, the elevated peripheral vascular resistance results from high levels of both norepinephrine and angiotensin II.

In hypertensive patients with pheochromocytoma, plasma volume is always reduced.

A statistically more important form of vasoconstrictive hypertension is that associated with renal artery stenosis. This type of arterial obstructive disease can be caused by either fibromuscular hyperplasia of the vessel wall or arteriosclerotic plaques. When a renal artery is first obstructed there is a rise in plasma renin activity and a subsequent increase in blood pressure. As the blood pressure rises there is some feedback supression of renin secretion. There is also a tendency for the hypoperfused kidney to retain salt. If the opposite kidney is normal the retained salt will be excreted and no volume expansion will occur. If, however, the opposite kidney is also underperfused, then salt will be retained, extracellular and plasma volumes will be expanded, and plasma renin activity will be suppressed. At this point the elevated blood pressure is sustained by the expanded volume rather than increased levels of angiotensin II.

In patients with chronic renal disease and renal insufficiency, extracellular and plasma volumes are expanded but plasma renin activity is not suppressed commensurate with the degree of volume expansion. In these patients the degree of hypertension correlates better with the product of plasma volume and plasma renin activity than with plasma volume alone. Inhibition of the formation or the action of angiotensin II in these patients will lower the blood pressure partially but not completely to normal, indicating some contribution of the renin-angiotensin system to the hypertension. These patients also have expanded plasma volumes and measurable levels of the Na^+-transport inhibitor in their plasma. Reduction of plasma volume by salt restriction, diuretics, or in some instances dialysis is an effective means of controlling the hypertension.

The great majority of patients have no identifiable cause for their hypertension and thus are said to have *essential hypertension*. Moreover, this form of hypertension does not fit into the pure volume-dependent or the pure vasoconstrictor forms of hypertension. Plasma renin activity is elevated in about 25 percent, is normal in about 50 percent, and is suppressed in about 25 percent of these patients. A widely held view is that an inherited defect in the kidney's ability to excrete dietary salt loads causes these patients to become volume expanded and hypertensive when ingesting the urban high-salt diets. However, these patients have an inverse rather than positive correlation between blood pressure and plasma volume; the higher the blood pressure, the smaller the plasma volume. Plasma volume is severely reduced in high-renin hypertension, is modestly reduced in normal renin-hypertension, and is near normal in low-renin hypertension. High levels of circulating Na^+-transport inhibitor have been reported in plasma of some hypertensive patients. In some studies the levels have been highest in low-renin hypertension, while in other studies the levels have correlated with the level of the blood pressure irrespective of the plasma renin activity. Low-renin hypertension does not respond well to inhibitors of the renin-angiotensin system, but usually shows a good response to salt restriction or diuretics. Thus, this form of essential hypertension shows some of the characteristics of volume-dependent hypertension. In contrast, high-renin hypertension usually shows good response to inhibition of the renin-angiotensin system, but shows no response (or even may worsen) to salt restriction or diuretics. This form, therefore, resembles pure vasoconstrictor hypertension. Normal-renin hypertension responds to both inhibition of the renin-angiotensin system and salt restriction or diuretics, and thus appears to be a mixed form of hypertension.

Diagnostic Workup. The goal of the initial workup of a hypertensive patient is to identify any treatable cause of the hypertension and also to evaluate the contribution of volume overload and circulating vasoconstrictors in the hypertensive process. A useful approach is to perform a urinalysis and measure blood urea nitrogen (BUN), plasma creatinine, potassium, and renin activity, and urine sodium and potassium while the patient is ingesting his or her normal diet and before starting any therapy. An abnormal urinalysis, BUN, or creatinine will identify those patients with renal disease. A low plasma potassium, high urine potassium (greater than 30 mEq/day), and low plasma renin activity indicates renal potassium wasting and volume expansion and thus suggests an excess of mineralocorticoid hormone. Such a patient should be further evaluated for primary hyperaldosteronism or Cushing's disease by measuring aldosterone and cortisol levels under appro-

"Essential" hypertension is that form of hypertension with no identifiable cause.

In hypertensive patients, abnormalities in BUN or plasma creatinine levels, and an abnormal urinalysis, indicate renal disease.

priate physiological conditions. In contrast, low potassium in both plasma and urine with a high plasma renin activity would suggest previous diuretic therapy. A high plasma renin activity with normal blood chemistries suggests previous treatment with birth control pills, renal vascular disease, high renin essential hypertension, or pheochromocytoma. Depending on the findings of the history and physical examination, these patients may be evaluated further with urinary catecholamines, renal angiograms, and/or renal venous plasma renin activities. Normal plasma renin activity and blood chemistries do not rule out renal artery disease, but usually represent normal renin essential hypertension and no further workup is indicated. All hypertensive patients should have a baseline electrocardiogram to evaluate for left ventricular strain and/or arrhythmias.

Treatment. Long-standing untreated hypertension may result in cerebral vascular accidents, myocardial hypertrophy and congestive heart failure, coronary artery disease, renal disease (nephrosclerosis), and accelerated or malignant hypertension. Lowering the blood pressure in hypertensive patients prevents the development of the malignant phase of hypertension and reduces the incidence of cerebral vascular accidents and nephrosclerosis, but has little effect on the cardiac complications. The most likely explanation for this latter dilemma is that treatment with salt restriction, diuretics, or vasodilators may induce a compensatory increase in sympathetic activity which in turn may have deleterious effects on the myocardium and coronary circulation.

The initial treatment for mild-to-moderate hypertension depends on whether the hypertension is primarily volume-dependent, vasoconstrictive, or mixed. Low-renin or volume-dependent hypertension should be treated with low-salt diet and/or diuretics, and usually does not require antirenin drugs. High-renin hypertension does not respond well to low-salt diet or diuretics, and is best treated with β-adrenergic antagonists to block renin secretion or, in more severe hypertension, with converting enzyme inhibitors to block angiotensin AII production. Normal-renin (or mixed) hypertension will usually require a combination of low-salt diet and/or diuretics plus a β-adrenergic antagonist. More severe forms of hypertension may require the use of a directly acting vasodilator. These drugs, however, invariably induce renal salt retention and sympathetic overactivity and always require the concurrent use of diuretics and β-adrenergic antagonists.

Severe forms of hypertension require treatment by directly acting vasodilator drugs.

REFERENCES

Seifter, J. L., Skorecki, K. L., Stivelman, J. C., Haupert, G., and Brenner, B. M.: Control of extracellular fluid volume and pathogenesis of edema formation. *In* Brenner, B. M., and Rector, F. C., Jr., eds.: The Kidney, 3rd Edition. W. B. Saunders Co., Philadelphia, 1986. *An in-depth review of the mechanisms that regulate extracellular fluid volume and edema formation.*

Reineck, H. J., and Stein, J. H.: Renal regulation of extracellular fluid volume. *In* Brenner, B. M., and Stein, J. H., eds.: Sodium and Water Homeostasis. Churchill Livingstone, Inc., New York, 1978. *A brief, but excellent review of extracellular volume regulation.*

Skorecki, K. L., and Brenner, B. M.: Body fluid homeostasis in congestive heart failure and cirrhosis with ascites. Am. J. Med. 72:323–338, 1982. *A thorough review of the mechanisms of edema formation in cirrhosis and nephrosis.*

Skorecki, K. L., Nadler, S. P., Badr, K. F., and Brenner, B. M.: Renal and systemic manifestations of glomerular disease. *In* Brenner, B. M., and Rector, F. C., Jr., eds.: The Kidney, 3rd Edition. W. B. Saunders Co., Philadelphia, 1986.
Includes a thorough discussion of the pathophysiology of edema formation in the nephrotic and nephritic syndromes.

Alpern, R. J.: Renal sodium retention in liver disease. West. J. Med. 138:852–860, 1983.
A defense of the classic theory of sodium retention in cirrhosis.

Anderson, R. J., and Linas, S. L.: Sodium depletion states. *In* Brenner, B. M., and Stein, J. H., eds.: Sodium and Water Homeostasis. Churchill Livingstone, Inc., New York, 1978.
A brief discussion of clinical conditions associated with depletion of extracellular fluid volume.

Coggins, C. H.: Nephrotic and nephritic edema. *In* Brenner, B. M., and Stein, J. H., eds.: Sodium and Water Homeostasis. Churchill Livingstone, Inc., New York, 1978.
A brief discussion of the mechanisms of edema formation in the nephrotic and nephritic syndromes.

Better, O. S., and Schrier, R. W.: Disturbed volume homeostasis in patients with cirrhosis of the liver. Kidney Int. 23:303–311, 1983.
A thorough review of the mechanisms of sodium retention in cirrhosis.

Kaplan, N. M.: Clinical Hypertension. Medcom Press, New York, 1973.
A simple, readable survey of hypertension, its causes and pathophysiology.

Laragh, J. H., Bühler, F., and Seldin, D. W., eds.: Frontiers in Hypertension Research. Springer-Verlag, New York, 1981.
Contains an excellent series of position papers summarizing current concepts of hypertension.

5

Acid-Base Homeostasis

NORMAL ACID-BASE HOMEOSTASIS

Acid continually enters body fluids and threatens maintenance of the blood's normal pH of 7.35 to 7.43. Intracellular and extracellular buffers and respiratory compensation can temporarily stabilize the pH when acid accumulates, but ultimately the kidney is responsible for ridding the body of excess acid. This chapter considers the sources of acid that enter body fluids, how partial defense of the blood pH is effected by buffering systems and respiration, and finally how the kidneys are able to dispose quantitatively of this acid while maintaining circulating buffer base (bicarbonate) at a constant level.

Sources of Endogenous Acids. While the lungs are capable of disposing of the large quantity of CO_2 (and hence carbonic acid) produced daily, *nonvolatile acid* must be excreted by the kidney. Such nonvolatile acids are derived from three sources: diet, intermediary metabolism, and stool base loss. Under normal conditions, approximately 70 mEq (1 mEq/kg of body weight) of acid are produced daily.

Diet. The usual, high-protein American diet contains amino acids and other substances that are potential acids. The chloride salt of lysine is metabolized to hydrochloric acid plus urea. Phosphoesters in proteins and nucleic acids can be hydrolyzed to form phosphoric acid. Sulfur-containing amino acids (methionine and cysteine) can be oxidized to generate sulfuric acid. Roughly 20 to 30 mEq of acid are derived daily from an average diet, proportional to protein intake.

Normal daily acid production is about 1 mEq/kg of body weight.

Metabolism. Incomplete oxidation of neutral foodstuffs such as glucose is normally responsible for the formation of about 20 to 30 mEq/day of organic acids. In some pathologic states, a large increase occurs in production of certain organic acids. Formation of *ketoacids* is increased in diabetes, alcoholism, or starvation. Similarly, toxin and drug ingestion can cause accelerated formation of organic acids (*formic acid* from methanol, *oxalic acid* from ethylene glycol, *salicylic acid* from aspirin). Another mechanism for increased endogenous acid production occurs if the hepatic conversion of *lactic acid* to glucose (the Cori cycle) is interrupted for any reason; because muscle produces such large amounts (750 to 1500 mEq/day), lactic acid will accumulate quickly. Thus, production of endogenous acids occurs normally but can also be increased by certain hormonal influences, by exogenous substrates, or by interruption of disposal pathways.

Stool. Normally about 20 to 30 mEq/day of bicarbonate or other equivalent base is lost in stools. In certain diarrheal diseases, base loss can be augmented tenfold. Base loss is equivalent to H^+ gain in the body fluids.

Body fluids are highly buffered to minimize changes in pH in the event of acid loading. Bicarbonate is the principal extracellular buffer.

Buffering Processes. If any of the above acids are added to an unbuffered solution, a rapid lowering of pH occurs. The body fluids, however, are highly buffered to minimize the change in pH that would otherwise ensue from an acid load. As shown in Figure 5–1, the principal extracellular buffer is *bicarbonate* (HCO_3^-), which is under physiologic regulation by the kidneys. In addition, intracellular buffers exist (proteins, hemoglobin, bone carbonates) that also participate in defending against an acid challenge. Indeed, over half of any H^+ added to the body reacts with intracellular rather than extracellular buffers. A proportionally greater role for intracellular buffers occurs as the acid load becomes larger and bicarbonate stores are depleted. Bicarbonate titrated by acid is converted to CO_2 and excreted by the lungs. Thus, two buffering responses occur when an acid (H^+) is added to intracellular (B^-) or extracellular (HCO_3^-) buffers.

$$H^+ + B^- \rightleftharpoons HB$$
$$H^+ + HCO_3^- \rightleftharpoons H_2CO_3 \rightleftharpoons CO_2 \uparrow + H_2O$$

These buffering reactions are rapid (requiring less than an hour), are efficient in tending to minimize the degree of acidemia (unless an overwhelming acid load is encountered), and are reversible (when HCO_3^- is regenerated by renal mechanisms). Renal HCO_3^- regeneration restores the basic intracellular buffer form (B^-) since hydrogen ions in all body fluid compartments are in a dynamic steady state.

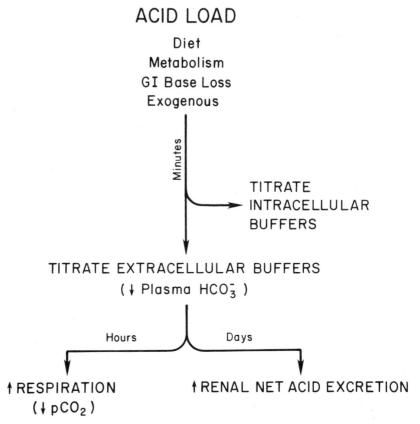

Figure 5–1. Response of intra- and extracellular buffers to an acid load.

Respiratory Compensation. The change in pH that would otherwise result from a change in HCO_3^- concentration is ameliorated by a parallel change in pCO_2. Since the *Henderson-Hasselbalch equation* states that

$$pH = 6.1 + \log \frac{[HCO_3^-]}{(.03 \times pCO_2)}$$

it follows that pH tends to be stabilized if pCO_2 varies with HCO_3^- concentration. The pCO_2 during metabolic acidosis decreases by 1.25 mm Hg per mEq/liter decrement in $[HCO_3^-]$. For example, the pCO_2 should change about 12.5 mm Hg (from 40 to 27.5 mm Hg) if the HCO_3^- concentration falls by 10 mEq/liter (from 24 to 14 mEq/liter). In so doing, the pH is only slightly depressed to 7.30, instead of 7.15 had there been no change in ventilation, i.e., if pCO_2 had remained at 40 mm Hg. The respiratory change induced by metabolic acidosis takes about 6 to 12 hours to complete.

A rise in pCO_2 during metabolic alkalosis also occurs. The pCO_2 increases by about 0.5 mm Hg per mEq/liter increment in HCO_3^- concentration. This response also takes several hours to develop. The hypoventilatory response to alkalemia eventually becomes overridden if hypoxia supervenes.

While the discussion so far has focused on the pulmonary adaptation to primary metabolic disorders, i.e., primary alterations in the blood HCO_3^- concentration, the converse compensatory changes also occur. That is, the kidneys lower blood HCO_3^- concentration if pCO_2 is chronically depressed and vice versa. These renal adjustments in HCO_3^- concentration take several days to develop. Thus a change in pCO_2 that occurs before renal compensation can be effected is termed an *acute respiratory disorder*. After renal compensation, it is called a *chronic respiratory disorder*.

In summary, a change in pCO_2 or in HCO_3^- concentration will induce a parallel change in the other. Such compensatory alterations tend to restore blood pH toward, but rarely completely back to, normal. It should not be inferred that it is the pH that is being sensed physiologically. Indeed, under certain circumstances, a "compensatory" adaptation can make the pH worse, not better. But the usual consequence of the respiratory and renal responses to each other is to stabilize the blood pH in simple acid-base disorders.

Renal Compensation. While the chemical buffering and respiratory responses to an acid challenge offer temporary defense of the blood pH, the ultimate responsibility for regenerating lost HCO_3^- and fully restoring acid-base homeostasis resides with the kidney. The kidney is actually faced with two problems. First, because of its high glomerular filtration rate (GFR), the kidney must reclaim all filtered HCO_3^- (normally about 4500 mEq daily). Not to do so would result in urinary HCO_3^- loss and would exacerbate the depletion of HCO_3^- already incurred by the buffering of metabolic acids. Second, HCO_3^- lost in titration by dietary and endogenous acid production must be regenerated. The kidney deals with these two problems separately, in two parts of the nephron.

HCO_3^- Reclamation. Of the 4500 mEq/day of HCO_3^- normally filtered, 80 to 90 percent is reabsorbed by the proximal convoluted tubule. As illustrated in Figure 5–2, HCO_3^- reabsorption is effected by H^+ secretion in a neutral exchange for Na^+. Luminal carbonic acid thus formed is broken down to CO_2 and water under the catalytic influence of carbonic anhydrase. The CO_2 can then diffuse back into the cell to be hydrated to carbonic acid under the catalytic influence of intracellular carbonic anhydrase. The carbonic acid in turn decomposes to form H^+ (to be used again for luminal secretion) and HCO_3^- which exits across the basolateral membrane and enters the blood.

The fraction of HCO_3^- reabsorbed in the proximal tubule is highly sensitive to changes in extracellular volume. This effect may be mediated, at least in part, by concurrent alterations in GFR. Extracellular volume depletion augments the fraction of HCO_3^- reabsorbed while volume expansion tends to suppress reabsorption. Potassium stores, parathyroid hormone, and acute changes in pCO_2 may also affect proximal HCO_3^- reabsorption but current evidence suggests that such effects are relatively small in the physiologic range of these parameters.

Although not pertinent to the discussion of the renal response to metabolic acidosis, it should be noted also that the proximal HCO_3^- reabsorptive capacity can be saturated. If the blood HCO_3^- concentration is raised above normal, for instance by HCO_3^- loading, there is no commensurate increase in proximal HCO_3^- reabsorption. The excess

Acute and chronic respiratory disorders are distinguished by whether the change in pCO_2 occurs before or after renal compensation is effected.

The proximal convoluted tubule reabsorbs 80 to 90 percent of the 4500 mEq of HCO_3^- normally filtered each day.

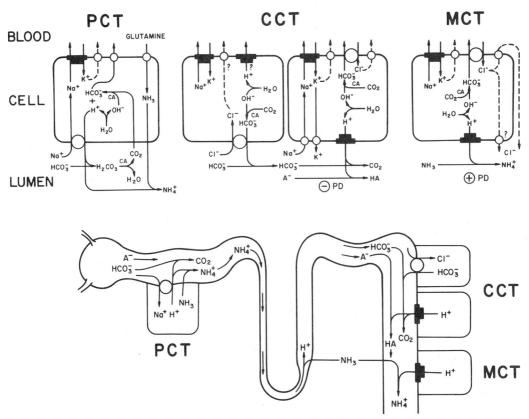

Figure 5–2. Acidification mechanisms in proximal nephron and distal nephron.

filtered HCO_3^- load will thereby cause an increase in delivery of HCO_3^- out of the proximal tubule, which will swamp the distal nephron's low capacity for HCO_3^- reabsorption and lead to urinary HCO_3^- excretion. The blood HCO_3^- concentration then returns to normal. By this mechanism, the proximal nephron normally protects the body from an elevation in the blood HCO_3^- concentration.

Net Acid Excretion—New HCO_3^- Generation. Once most of the filtered HCO_3^- is reabsorbed by the proximal nephron, the process by which new HCO_3^- is created can take place in the distal nephron (distal convoluted tubule, cortical and medullary collecting tubules). The distal nephron secretes H^+ formed into the lumen, but not in direct exchange for Na^+, as was the case in the proximal nephron. The mechanism appears to be an *electrogenic proton-translocating ATPase* which can be directly stimulated by aldosterone. In addition, aldosterone-dependent electrogenic Na^+ reabsorption in the cortical collecting tubule creates a lumen-negative potential. This more favorable electrochemical gradient stimulates H^+ secretion secondarily. By means of such electrogenic H^+ secretion, the cortical collecting tubule first reabsorbs whatever HCO_3^- escaped proximal reabsorption. The luminal pH can then be reduced to very low levels, less than 5.5. As seen in Figure 5–2, the low luminal pH allows titration of filtered non-bicarbonate buffers (A^-) with relatively high pKa, such as phosphate ($HPO_4^=$) and creatinine. Thus, phosphate is titrated by H^+ secretion.

$$H^+ + HPO_4^= \rightarrow H_2PO_4^-$$

The HCO_3^- generated in the cell diffuses into the blood, while $H_2PO_4^-$ is excreted into the urine. Buffers capable of being titrated in the pH range achievable in the lumen of the distal nephron (about 4.5 to 5.5) are called *titratable acids*.

HCO_3^- generated in the cell diffuses into the blood, while H_2PO_4^- is excreted into the urine.

If the conjugate anions of all dietary ingested acid were capable of being reacidified by the kidney, HCO_3^- would be regenerated quantitatively and acid-base equilibrium re-established. However, many ingested acids have a very low pKa (e.g., sulfuric or hydrochloric acid) and the conjugate anion cannot be acidified at a urinary pH even as low as 4.5. The kidney compensates for these untitratable anions by creating a new buffer, *ammonia* (NH_3), by hydrolysis of glutamine. Ammonia is produced in the proximal tubule and is trapped in the proximal lumen as NH_4^+ until it reaches the bend of the loop of Henle. It is then released as NH_3 to diffuse into the acid lumen of the medullary collecting tubule, where it reacts with H^+ to form the nondiffusible *ammonium* (NH_4^+) which is excreted in the urine. The lower the urinary pH, the more NH_3, trapping as NH_4^+, is formed at any given level of luminal pH.

The cortical collecting tubule also has a transport mechanism capable of secreting bicarbonate in exchange for chloride. Bicarbonate secretion would tend to antagonize the acidification processes discussed above, but its quantitative significance is unknown. This mechanism may play an important role in helping to correct metabolic alkalosis.

Thus, the distal nephron regenerates blood HCO_3^- by secreting H^+ into the lumen to lower the pH and thereby to form titratable acids and NH_4^+. Titratable acid and NH_4^+ excretion (minus any residual urinary HCO_3^-) is termed *net acid excretion*. Urinary net acid excretion in a steady state creates an amount of new HCO_3^- daily (about 1 mEq/kg) equivalent to the HCO_3^- lost by dietary, metabolic, or stool acid production.

The distal nephron normally adjusts the amount of new HCO_3^- generated (the amount of net acid excreted), to equal that of acid generated. It also has the ability to increase acid excretion if extra acid loads occur. A several-fold increase in net acid excretion can occur in *ketoacidosis* (by an increase in titratable acid production) or in chronic hydrochloric acid loading (by augmentation of ammoniagenesis and hence NH_4^+ excretion). Besides adapting to acid input, distal acidification is also very sensitive to Na^+ delivery and to circulating aldosterone levels. The ability to secrete H^+ is diminished if distal Na^+ delivery is severely curtailed or in hypoaldosteronemic states.

In summary, the proximal nephron reabsorbs most of the filtered HCO_3^- and represents a high capacity, saturable, extracellular volume-sensitive process. The distal nephron generates new HCO_3^- by lowering the luminal pH for titration of filtered ($HPO_4^=$) or endogenous (NH_3) buffers and represents a large pH-gradient, low capacity system sensitive to aldosterone and electrogenic Na^+ transport. It is important to remember that H^+ secretion mediates both proximal and distal acidification processes.

H^+ secretion mediates both proximal and distal acidification processes.

Proximal nephron function is evaluated by the ability to reabsorb

HCO_3^- quantitatively until the blood HCO_3^- exceeds a normal level of about 24 to 26 mEq/liter. Distal nephron function is evaluated by the ability to generate a low urinary pH (less than 5.5) during spontaneous or induced acidosis and to increase titratable acid and NH_4^+ excretion to values greater than 25 and 40 μEq/min, respectively.

DIAGNOSIS OF ACID-BASE DISORDERS

Suspicion that an acid-base disorder exists arises usually on clinical grounds or by the discovery of an abnormal blood pH, pCO_2, or HCO_3^- concentration. In evaluating acid-base data, it is necessary to: (1) verify that the values are correct; (2) assign a primary diagnostic category to the disorder; (3) ascertain whether the proper physiologic pulmonary or renal compensatory processes have occurred; and (4) then specifically identify the acid-base derangement using other laboratory (e.g., anion gap, plasma K^+ concentration, urinary electrolytes) and clinical information.

Verification of Acid-Base Parameters. It follows from the mass action relationship of blood H^+ concentration, pCO_2, and HCO_3^- concentration:

$$H^+ + HCO_3^- \rightleftharpoons H_2CO_3 \rightleftharpoons H_2O + CO_2$$

that the *Henderson equation* is:

$$[H^+] = K \frac{(\alpha\ pCO_2)}{[HCO_3^-]}$$

where K is the carbonic acid dissociation constant and α is the solubility coefficient for CO_2 in blood. If it is remembered that $K \cdot \alpha$ is 24, then the relationship simplifies to: $[H^+] = \dfrac{24\ (pCO_2)}{[HCO_3^-]}$

The normal H^+ concentration is 40 nM (remembered as the last two digits of the normal pH of 7.40) and changes reciprocally by 1 nM for each change in pH of 0.01. The normal equality would be represented by:

$$40 = \frac{24\ (40)}{24}$$

The utility of this equation is exemplified by the following example. To calculate the HCO_3^- concentration for an arterial blood pH of 7.30 ($[H^+]$ = 50 nM) and pCO_2 of 25 mm Hg, the equation could be written as:

$$[HCO_3^-] = \frac{24 \times pCO_2}{[H^+]} = \frac{24 \times 25}{50} = 12\ \text{mmol}$$

The Henderson equation or its logarithmic transformation, the Henderson-Hasselbalch equation, is used to calculate the third acid-base value when only two are given or to verify that three given values are mutually compatible. The *Henderson-Hasselbalch equation* is:

$$pH = 6.1 + \log \frac{[HCO_3^-]}{(0.03 \times pCO_2)}$$

Nomenclature. Metabolic acid-base disturbances are classified as conditions in which there is a primary increase or decrease in HCO_3^- concentration secondary to addition or loss of nonvolatile acids or alkali to or from the extracellular fluid. Respiratory acid-base disturbances are those in which there is a primary change in arterial pCO_2, reflecting a primary increase or decrease in alveolar ventilation relative to existing CO_2 production. In general, simple uncomplicated metabolic or respiratory acidosis is associated with a decreased blood pH, while simple uncomplicated metabolic or respiratory alkalosis is associated with an increased blood pH. However, simultaneous occurrence of two or more acid-base disturbances can distort these more simple relationships and result in a wide range of pH values, depending on the relative importance of each of the underlying acid-base disturbances.

Simple metabolic (or respiratory) acidosis shows decreased blood pH, while simple metabolic (or respiratory) alkalosis shows increased blood pH.

The physiologic respiratory or renal response to a primary metabolic or chronic respiratory acid-base disturbance, respectively, is called *compensatory*. If there is a failure of a compensatory response to occur, then a separate disorder exists.

Acid-Base Map. Once a set of values for pH, P_{CO_2} and HCO_3^- concentration is obtained, the next step is to consult an acid-base map (Fig. 5–3). The shaded areas represent the 95 percent confidence limits of the six simple acid-base disorders. The appropriate respiratory compensations that occur in the two metabolic disorders are assumed to have fully occurred (which take 6 to 12 hours). It is further assumed that the metabolic (renal) adjustments in the plasma HCO_3^- concentration have not occurred in the acute respiratory disorders but have fully occurred in the chronic respiratory disorders (which takes 3 to 5 days). There are obviously intermediate temporal adjustments that are unrepresented on the nomogram.

If a set of acid-base values falls in a shaded area, the presumption is that a simple acid-base disorder exists. Sets of acid-base values that fall outside these areas imply either that sufficient time has not elapsed for the appropriate respiratory or renal compensation to occur or that a mixed (two or more disorders) acid-base disturbance exists. It is possible, however, that two disorders may combine so that the resulting set of values falls in the area of yet another disorder or even in the normal area. Clinical and laboratory clues often provide enough information to indicate that such a situation has occurred.

Anion Gap. A helpful piece of information when subcategorizing the metabolic acidoses and diagnosing mixed acid-base disorders is the anion gap. The plasma anion gap = $Na^+ - (HCO_3^- + Cl^-)$.

The anion gap is, technically, unmeasured cations subtracted from unmeasured anions.

The normal anion gap is 12 mEq/liter (range of 8 to 16 mEq/liter) and, for practical purposes, predominantly represents *albumin*, a polyanionic macromolecule. Technically the anion gap is actually the unmeasured anions minus unmeasured cations. For instance, a low anion gap is sometimes found in multiple myeloma when an excessive amount of cationic globulins contributes to the ionic composition of the

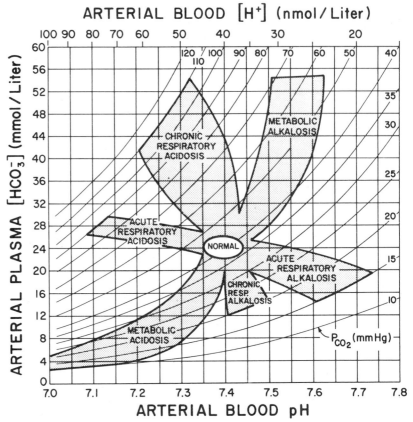

Figure 5–3. Acid-base nomogram.

blood. In practice, however, an elevation in the anion gap occurs in only two circumstances. First, the anion gap rises modestly when the negative charge density on albumin is increased in metabolic alkalosis. The reaction

$$H^+ + Albumin^- \rightleftharpoons H{\cdot}Albumin$$

is driven to the left in metabolic alkalosis. The charge on each albumin molecule is increased.

More important, the anion gap is elevated when an acid other than hydrochloric is added to the blood. In such a case, HCO_3^- is titrated and exhaled as CO_2 while the sodium salt of the conjugate anion of the acid remains in the blood. This conjugate anion is not routinely measured (since it is neither HCO_3^- nor Cl^-):

$$H^+ Anion^- + NaHCO_3 + NaCl \rightarrow H_2O$$
$$+ CO_2 \uparrow + Na^+ Anion^- + NaCl$$

The pre-existing Na^+ and Cl^- concentrations remain unchanged. Thus, the decrement in the HCO_3^- concentration is proportional to the rise in anion gap. The anion gap, in turn, is equal to the magnitude of the added unmeasured anion. Such an acidosis is termed a *high anion gap* or *normochloremic metabolic acidosis*. For instance, if 10 mM of an acid, HA, were added to normal blood, the HCO_3^- concentration would decrease by 10 mM, while the normal anion gap (X) of 12 mM would rise by 10 mM:

$$\text{Normal: } \underset{24}{NaHCO_3} + \underset{104}{NaCl} + \underset{12}{NaX} \qquad \text{Anion Gap} = X = 12$$

$$+ \underset{10}{HA} \rightarrow \underset{14}{NaHCO_3} + \underset{104}{NaCl} + \underset{12}{NaX} + \underset{10}{NaA} \qquad \text{Anion Gap} = X + A = 22$$

Conversely, if the acid added to the blood were equivalent to HCl, the fall in HCO_3^- concentration would be matched by a reciprocal rise in the Cl^- concentration. No change in anion gap would occur. Such an acidosis is termed a *normal anion gap* or *hyperchloremic metabolic acidosis*. For example, if 10 mM HCl or its metabolic equivalent were added to the blood, the anion gap (X) would remain unchanged from 12 mM:

$$\text{Normal: } \underset{24}{NaHCO_3} + \underset{104}{NaCl} + \underset{12}{NaX} \qquad \text{Anion Gap} = X = 12$$

$$+ \underset{10}{HCl} \rightarrow \underset{14}{NaHCO_3} + \underset{114}{NaCl} + \underset{12}{NaX} \qquad \text{Anion Gap} = X = 12$$

The presence of an anion gap therefore signifies that a nonhydrochloric acid has been added to the blood. In practice, such acids are few, as will be discussed subsequently. The differential diagnosis is thus simplified.

The presence of an anion gap signifies that a nonhydrochloric acid has been added to the blood.

METABOLIC ACIDOSIS

As shown in Figure 5–4, a low bicarbonate concentration should first be evaluated using arterial blood gases and the acid-base nomogram to verify that a metabolic acidosis exists. The anion gap will then serve to differentiate the two subgroups composing metabolic acidosis.

Normal Anion Gap. A normal anion gap (hyperchloremic) metabolic acidosis may be attributable to: (1) rapid dilution of plasma HCO_3^- by saline (dilution acidosis); (2) addition of large quantities of HCl (or its equivalent, as in hyperalimentation) to the body fluids; (3) addition of an acid other than HCl with subsequent titration of HCO_3^- and rapid renal excretion of the accompanying anion and replacement by Cl^- (e.g., recovery from ketoacidosis); (4) HCO_3^- loss from the body fluids from the gastrointestinal tract with Cl^- retention; or (5) defective renal acidification with renal loss of the conjugate base and Cl^- retention. The last two mechanisms, gastrointestinal alkali loss and renal acidification defects, are by far the most common causes of a normal anion gap metabolic acidosis.

Gastrointestinal Bicarbonate Loss. Accelerated loss of alkaline fluid, as diarrhea or pancreatic or biliary drainage, will cause H^+ accumulation in the body fluids. Chloride is retained directly (as the result of gut HCO_3^-/Cl^- countertransport) or indirectly, by renal mechanisms responsive to the resultant extracellular volume contrac-

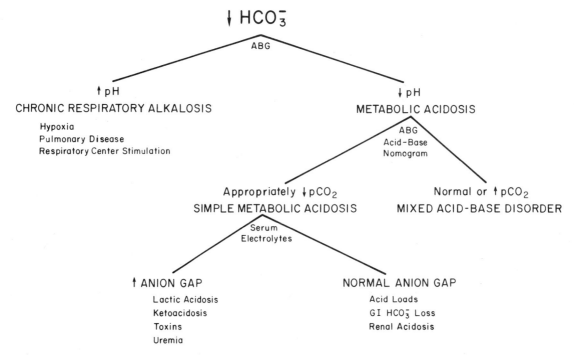

Figure 5–4. Differential diagnosis and approach to a decreased plasma HCO_3^- concentration. ABG, arterial blood gas determination.

tion. Volume contraction also produces hypokalemia because of direct gastrointestinal loss plus urinary loss secondary to hyperreninemic hyperaldosteronism. Urinary net acid excretion, primarily as NH_4^+, is high in an attempt to repair the acidosis.

Renal Acidoses. Defects in the various steps of normal renal acidification can produce a hyperchloremic acidosis even though dietary metabolic and gastrointestinal acid production is not increased. As summarized in Table 5–1, the defects include an inability to reabsorb HCO_3^- (proximal renal tubular acidosis) or an inability to excrete sufficient net acid. The failure of the distal nephron to excrete net acid may be caused by: (1) an isolated defect in lowering the urinary pH (classical distal renal tubular acidosis); (2) a total failure of the H^+ and K^+ secretory function of the distal nephron (generalized distal renal

Table 5–1. HYPERCHLOREMIC METABOLIC ACIDOSES

	Renal Defect	Plasma $[K^+]$	Proximal Acidification HCO_3^- Reabsorption (HCO_3^- Loading)	Distal Acidification	
				UpH_{min} (Acidosis)	$U_{NH_4^+}V + U_{TA}V$ (Acidosis)
Gastrointestinal HCO_3^- Loss	None	↓	Nl	≤ 5.5	↑
Renal Acidoses					
Proximal	↓ Proximal acidification	↓	↓	< 5.5	Nl
Classical distal	↓ Distal pH gradient	↓	Nl	> 5.5	↓
Generalized distal	↓ Aldosterone action	↑	Nl	< 5.5	↓
Glomerular insufficiency	↓ NH_3 production	Nl	Nl	< 5.5	↓

Nl, normal; TA, titratable acid.

tubular acidosis); or (3) the failure to excrete sufficient NH_4^+ (renal tubular acidosis of renal insufficiency).

When proximal Na^+/H^+ countertransport is disordered, or carbonic anhydrase is inhibited, *proximal renal tubular acidosis (RTA)* (also called type II RTA) results. The acidification defect usually occurs in association with the urinary wastage of other Na^+ co-transported substances in the proximal tubule such as glucose, amino acids, phosphorus, and uric acid (Fanconi's syndrome). Excessive delivery of $NaHCO_3$ out of the proximal tubule to the distal tubule also results in enhanced K^+ secretion and hypokalemia. During acidosis, the filtered HCO_3^- load is reduced to an extent that delivery of HCO_3^- out of the proximal tubule is only slightly above normal and the distal nephron can compensate for any slight excess. Consequently, the distal nephron can lower urine pH and produce net acid normally. However, if the blood HCO_3^- and filtered HCO_3^- load is returned to normal values, delivery of HCO_3^- out of the proximal tubule increases, the relatively low-capacity distal nephron is completely overwhelmed and massive bicarbonaturia (>15 percent of the filtered load) results. This form of RTA is rare and usually ascribable to multiple myeloma, genetic defects (cystinosis, Wilson's disease), heavy metals (lead, mercury, cadmium), drugs that inhibit carbonic anhydrase (acetazolamide), and some secondary hyperparathyroid/vitamin D-deficient states. Bone disease is commonly found. Treatment rests in administering large amounts of bicarbonate and potassium. Volume contraction by diuretics can be used to stimulate fractional proximal HCO_3^- reabsorption.

Fanconi's syndrome is the name given to a group of conditions, either hereditary or acquired, with characteristic disorders of proximal tubule function.

The inability of the distal nephron to lower the luminal pH and hence titrate buffers is called *classical distal RTA* (also called type I RTA). Since H^+ secretion is defective, distal K^+ secretion is accelerated and results in hypokalemia as Na^+ is reabsorbed. The diagnosis of this form of RTA is confirmed when a urinary pH greater than 5.5 with deficient urinary acid excretion is found. Normal proximal HCO_3^- reabsorption is present even when filtered HCO_3^- concentrations are raised to a normal level. Nephrocalcinosis and nephrolithiasis are common, either as a cause or a result of classical distal RTA. Other etiologic factors include autoimmune diseases (Sjögren's syndrome, lupus), drugs (amphotericin B) and tubulointerstitial diseases. Treatment consists of providing enough base, usually as $NaHCO_3$ or Na · citrate, to compensate for daily acid production (about 1 mEq/day).

Functional hypoaldosteronism can occur from a variety of causes and gives rise to a *generalized distal RTA* (also called type IV RTA) in which the secretion of both H^+ and K^+ in the distal nephron is impaired. In this disorder(s) the hyperchloremic acidosis is associated with hyperkalemia. This common form of RTA may result from: (1) defective adrenal synthesis of aldosterone (adrenal destruction, enzymatic defects); (2) defective release of aldosterone secondary to hyporeninemia (diabetes, tubulointerstitial diseases); or (3) distal nephron damage and hence end-organ insensitivity to high levels of aldosterone (tubulointerstitial disease). Although the ability to lower urinary pH remains intact, the quantitative amount of H^+ and K^+ secreted is subnormal. The associated hyperkalemia also suppresses renal NH_3 synthesis, exacerbating the acidification defect. Treatment consists of replacing mineralocorticoid when deficient or lowering K^+ by diet, diuretics, or ion-exchange resins.

At a glomerular filtration rate of about 20 to 30 ml/min, the *RTA of glomerular insufficiency* often appears. In this *normokalemic* RTA, insufficient NH_4^+ is excreted to maintain normal net acid excretion. Treatment is base ($NaHCO_3$) therapy equivalent to daily acid production.

Elevated Anion Gap. *Lactic Acidosis.* Lactic acidosis results from increased lactic acid production from muscles or diminished conversion of lactic acid to glucose by the liver. Lactic acid overproduction is found in seizures or severe exercise. Insufficient use of lactic acid, which is more common, occurs in hypoxemia or states of poor tissue perfusion such as shock. The basic tenet of therapy for most forms of acute lactic acidosis is to repair the condition that has resulted in poor hepatic use of lactic acid.

Alcoholic ketoacidosis is treated with glucose-containing intravenous fluids.

Ketoacidosis. The three common forms of ketoacidosis include *diabetic; alcoholic*, after binge drinking; and *starvation*, in which ketone production is physiologically enhanced to provide substrate for brain and to spare endogenous protein degradation. The nitroprusside reaction for ketone detection measures only aceto-acetate and may be negative if the β-hydroxybutyrate/aceto-acetate ratio is high because of the altered intracellular redox state. This is often the case in alcoholic ketoacidosis. Therapy can be effected with insulin in the diabetic form, glucose-containing intravenous fluids (without insulin) in the alcoholic form, carbohydrate re-feeding in the starvation form, and rehydration in all forms.

Toxins. Various drugs and toxins can increase endogenous acid production. *Methanol* is sometimes ingested in place of ethanol (moonshine) and is metabolized to formic acid. Abdominal pain, nausea, vomiting, and visual disturbances including blindness result. An osmolar gap, the difference in the calculated osmolality ($2 \times Na$ + glucose/18 + BUN/2.8) and the measured osmolality, is sometimes found. This clue to the diagnosis results from the accumulation in blood of the low-molecular-weight methanol (32 daltons). Treatment consists of ethanol administration to inhibit methanol metabolism. Dialysis is sometimes necessary.

Ingestion of *ethylene glycol*, found in antifreeze, results in neurologic symptoms, cardiorespiratory collapse, and renal failure. Recognition of oxalate (the metabolite of ethylene glycol) crystals in the urine can aid in early diagnosis. An osmolar gap may also occur because of the low molecular weight (62 daltons) of ethylene glycol. Treatment is similar to that for methanol toxicity.

Poisoning with *salicylate* produces an anion gap acidosis in addition to a respiratory alkalosis. The responsible acids include salicylic acid as well as lactic acid. Tinnitus, nausea, vomiting, and shock can occur. Alkalinization of the blood and urine and sometimes dialysis are required for therapy.

A GFR of less than 20 ml/min results in failure to filter or excrete organic acids sufficiently.

Uremic Acidosis. When glomerular filtration rate falls below about 20 ml/min, organic and other conjugate anions of acids cannot be filtered and excreted in sufficient quantities. The resulting acidosis from accumulated organic acids is rarely severe. Before renal insufficiency progresses to the point that this acidosis supervenes, the hyperchloremic, normal anion gap RTA mentioned previously may predominate.

Symptoms and Treatment. Acidosis causes an increase in respiration, especially end-tidal volume (Kussmaul respiration), arterial vasodilation but venoconstriction, a fall in cardiac output (when arterial pH falls below 7.1), central nervous system depression, and a shift of the oxyhemoglobin dissociation curve to the right acutely and to the left chronically. Therapy is aimed at removing the cause of an acute acidosis. Primary indications for bicarbonate therapy include significant hyperkalemia or acidemia (pH less than about 7.10). Adverse effects of alkali therapy include hyperosmolality, hypokalemia, a rebound alkalosis, and perhaps exacerbation of lactic acidosis under some circumstances. In severe acidosis, the apparent volume of bicarbonate distribution may rise from the normal 50 percent of body weight to 100 percent because of the disproportionate contribution of intracellular buffers. When there is renal failure, hemodialysis can be used to remove lactate and administer bicarbonate. In such an event, the dialysate must contain bicarbonate rather than the usual base-equivalent acetate since the ability by the liver to convert acetate to bicarbonate is usually impaired in most organic acidoses. In lactic acidosis, the administration of dichloracetate has been proposed to increase hepatic lactate uptake and use, but the clinical efficacy of such treatment has not yet been established.

METABOLIC ALKALOSIS

As illustrated in Figure 5–5, a high HCO_3^- concentration and low Cl^- concentration represents either a chronic respiratory acidosis or metabolic alkalosis. Arterial blood gases, to document alkalinity, and

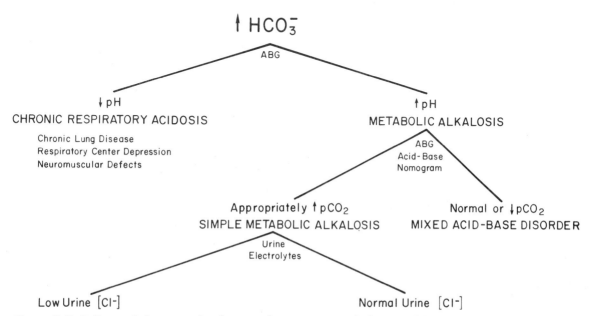

Figure 5–5. Differential diagnosis of and approach to an increased plasma HCO_3^- concentration. ABG, arterial blood gas determination.

Table 5–2. GENERATION OF METABOLIC ALKALOSIS

Source	Clinical Examples
Exogenous base administration	
Bicarbonate	$NaHCO_3$ therapy of acidosis
Carbonate	Antacids/milk-alkali syndrome
Acetate	Hyperalimentation
Citrate	Transfusions
GI acid loss	
Gastric	Vomiting/nasogastric suction
Stool	Congenital chloridorrhea
Urinary acid loss	
↑ Tubule flow rate/Na^+ delivery	Diuretics
↑ Mineralocorticoid activity	Hyperreninemic states
	Extracellular volume contraction
	Magnesium deficiency
	Bartter's syndrome
	Primary hypermineralocorticoid states
	Primary hyperaldosteronism
	Cushing's syndrome
	Adreno-genital syndromes
↑ Tubule lumen negativity	Nonreabsorbable anions (ketones, carbenicillin)
↑ pCO_2	Post-hypercapnia
? ↓ PTH/↑ Ca^{++}	Hypoparathyroidism/hypercalcemic states

Metabolic alkalosis has two phases: generation, with its HCO_3^- addition or H^+ removal, and renal maintenance of high HCO_3^- concentration.

the acid-base nomogram, to assess the appropriate degree of hypoventilation, will confirm the diagnosis of a simple metabolic alkalosis.

When assessing a patient with metabolic alkalosis, two questions must be asked: (1) What was the source of alkali that generated the alkalosis? and (2) What are the renal mechanisms that are operating to sustain the alkalosis? Answers to both questions are important in diagnosing and treating the disorder.

The first phase of metabolic alkalosis is the generation component (Table 5–2). In this phase, there is HCO_3^- addition to the body (base therapy), or, equivalently, H^+ removal from the stomach (vomiting, nasogastric aspiration), or loss in the urine (diuretics, hypermineralocorticoidism). Differentiation of these cases of metabolic alkalosis can often be achieved from the history and physical examination.

The second phase of metabolic alkalosis involves the renal maintenance of the high HCO_3^- concentration. The kidney normally quantitatively excretes excess HCO_3^- and thereby prevents the blood HCO_3^- from exceeding normal values. But the kidney in metabolic alkalosis is "reset" so that a HCO_3^- diuresis does not occur despite an elevated blood HCO_3^- concentration. In fact, the urine is acid, the so-called "parodoxical aciduria" of metabolic alkalosis.

There are three mechanisms proposed to account for the "resetting" of renal HCO_3^- reabsorption in the setting of a high blood HCO_3^- concentration (Table 5–3). First, GFR may be depressed (by intrinsic renal disease, extracellular volume depletion, or perhaps K^+ depletion) so that filtered HCO_3^- load remains normal despite a high blood HCO_3^- concentration. Normal rates of renal H^+ secretion then suffice to reabsorb all filtered HCO_3^- and sustain the alkalosis. Second, if the GFR remains normal so that the filtered HCO_3^- concentration and load increase, it has been suggested that the accompanying extracellular

**Table 5–3. POTENTIAL RENAL MECHANISMS RESPONSIBLE FOR
MAINTAINING METABOLIC ALKALOSIS**

Arterial [HCO_3^-]	GFR	Filtered HCO_3^- Load	Absolute Proximal HCO_3^- Reabsorption	Absolute Distal HCO_3^- Reabsorption	Urinary HCO_3^-
↑	↓	Nl	Nl	Nl	0
↑	Nl	↑	↑	Nl	0
↑	Nl	↑	Nl	↑	0

Nl, normal.

volume contraction (Cl^- depletion) and K^+ depletion stimulate proximal nephron acidification. Enhanced proximal acidification would prevent excess HCO_3^- delivery to the distal nephron and thereby prevent bicarbonaturia. Finally, high mineralocorticoid levels found in some forms of metabolic alkalosis (primary hyperaldosteronism) might be capable of augmenting the usually minimal distal acidifying capacity to reabsorb the increased filtered HCO_3^- load. The proximal nephron in this case would have a stable or even reduced (from volume expansion) HCO_3^- reabsorptive capacity. Other factors that can potentiate the effect by mineralocorticoids to stimulate distal acidification include increased flow and Na^+ to distal sites, nonreabsorbable anions, potassium deficiency, and hypercapnia.

The most useful clinical classification of metabolic alkalosis distinguishes two groups. This grouping is based on the above pathophysiologic mechanisms responsible for maintaining the alkalosis (Fig. 5–6). In general, if extracellular volume depletion has caused a reduction in GFR and/or a stimulation of proximal reabsorption, there will be a low urine Cl^- concentration, usually less than 10 mEq/liter (unless a renal Cl^- reabsorptive defect concurrently exists as with diuretics or Bartter's syndrome). Such alkaloses respond to saline therapy because extracellular volume repletion corrects the factors that maintain the alkalosis. Conversely, alkaloses without volume depletion are usually maintained by enhanced distal acidification. These alkaloses often manifest signs of extracellular volume overload (hypertension) and will obviously be unresponsive to further volume expansion by saline. There must be specific correction of the factors stimulating distal acidification to repair these alkaloses.

Bartter's syndrome is a primary juxtaglomerular cell hyperplasia with secondary hyperaldosteronism, found in children with hypokalemic alkalosis.

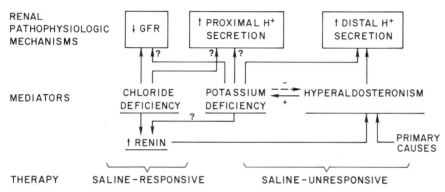

Figure 5–6. Metabolic alkalosis, its mechanisms, mediators, and responses to saline therapy.

Table 5–4. TREATMENT OF METABOLIC ALKALOSIS

	Saline-Responsive	Saline-Resistant
Laboratory Features	Low urinary Cl⁻ High aldosterone	High urinary Cl⁻ High aldosterone

Clinical Examples	Normotensive
	  Bicarbonate therapy of
	    organic acidosis
	  Vomiting/nasogastric
	    suction
	  Diuretics
	  Post-hypercapnia
		Hypertensive
		  Primary aldosteronism
		  Cushing's syndrome
		  Renal artery stenosis
		  Renal failure plus alkali
		    therapy
		
		Normotensive
		  Magnesium deficiency
		  Severe potassium deficiency
		  Bartter's syndrome

Saline-Responsive Alkalosis. These alkaloses usually involve simultaneous H^+ and Cl^- loss from the stomach (vomiting, nasogastric aspiration) or from the kidney (diuretics, hypercapnia). The H^+ loss generates the alkalosis while the Cl^- loss, equivalent to extracellular volume depletion, maintains it. Therapy with saline alone is sufficient to repair the alkalosis but concurrent K^+ deficits should also be repaired. These alkaloses are summarized in Table 5–4.

Removing HCl from the stomach is equivalent to adding $NaHCO_3$ to the blood.

Gastrointestinal HCO_3^- Loss. HCl removal from the stomach is equivalent to $NaHCO_3$ addition to the blood. Initially, the rise in plasma HCO_3^- concentration causes an appropriate alkaline diuresis. However, after about a day, the extracellular volume depletion is sensed by the kidney and the fractional HCO_3^- reabsorptive capacity is increased. The high plasma HCO_3^- concentration then no longer causes a HCO_3^- diuresis and the urine reverts to being acidic. At this point, daily acid production equals urinary net acid excretion and the metabolic alkalosis is sustained. Thus, following the generation of a metabolic alkalosis, the renal maintenance phase has two components: an initial alkaline diuresis that is followed by complete HCO_3^- retention with an acid urine. If vomiting or nasogastric aspiration recurs, the alkaline diuresis ($NaHCO_3$ or $KHCO_3$) will also transiently reappear. K^+ losses are mediated almost exclusively by the kidney. Urinary K^+ wastage (there is very little K^+ in gastric contents) results from hyperreninemic hyperaldosteronism induced by volume depletion. For the same reasons, the urine is free of Cl^-. Saline reverses the pathophysiologic sequence to restore acid-base normality. K^+ should also be repleted.

Diuretics. The most common cause of enhanced net acid excretion is the use of diuretics, especially loop and thiazide diuretics. Both cause accelerated NaCl delivery to the distal cation exchange sites. The increased luminal flow rate and Na^+ delivery accelerates distal Na^+ reabsorption, magnifies the luminal negative potential difference, and hence stimulates H^+ and K^+ secretion. The increased plasma HCO_3^- concentration is generated by the augmented urinary net acid excretion as well as by extracellular volume depletion, which concentrates the remaining amount of HCO_3^- (contraction alkalosis). The metabolic alkalosis is maintained by the continued high distal acidification rates, amplified by the volume contraction–induced hyperaldosteronism, in addition to enhanced fractional proximal HCO_3^- reabsorption caused by the extracellular volume depletion. The urine will contain Cl^- if diuretics continue to be administered, unless the extracellular volume depletion becomes severe and GFR is significantly depressed. Withdrawal of diuretics will stop the H^+, Cl^-, and K^+ losses. Extracellular volume repletion is necessary to restore the normal renal response to a high blood HCO_3^- concentration. HCO_3^- diuresis will not occur until Cl^- deficits are repaired.

Post-hypercapnia. In chronic respiratory acidosis, distal acidification is stimulated and a high HCO_3^- concentration results. Cl^- loss also occurs as a result of the direct effects of hypercapnia and can be exaggerated if diuretics are used. If the pCO_2 is then normalized, the kidney will quantitatively excrete the excess HCO_3^- unless significant extracellular volume depletion is present due to the pre-existing Cl^- loss. Metabolic alkalosis then results. Recurrent periods of hypercapnia followed by normocapnia will exacerbate the renal H^+ and Cl^- losses and make the metabolic alkalosis worse. Liberalization of salt intake plus discontinuation of diuretics allows normalization of the blood HCO_3^- concentration.

Saline-Resistant Alkalosis. These uncommon disorders are usually a consequence of primary hypermineralocorticoidism (primary aldosteronism or excessive ingestion of licorice, which contains a mineralocorticoid). Increased distal nephron acidification generates and then maintains the alkalosis despite the extracellular volume expansion and hypertension. Excessive alkali intake with a diminished GFR (milk-alkali syndrome) results in the same picture with a normal or expanded extracellular volume and the presence of urinary Cl^-. Primary hyperreninism, not driven by extracellular volume depletion, also occurs in a few renal disorders (Bartter's syndrome, renal artery stenosis, Mg^{++} deficiency). These alkaloses are summarized in Table 5–4.

Symptoms and Treatment. Metabolic alkalosis causes changes in peripheral and central nervous system function similar to those seen in hypocalcemia: mental confusion and obtundation, a predisposition to seizures, parasthesias, cramping and tetany. There can be aggravation of arrhythmias and hypoxemia in pulmonary disease. Related problems due to common coexistent electrolyte disorders such as hypokalemia and hypophosphatemia also frequently arise. Treatment is aimed at removing the source of the excess alkali and the factors contributing to the renal maintenance of the high HCO_3^- concentration as outlined above. In renal failure, dialysis against a dialysate with a low concentration of base (HCO_3^- or acetate) can be employed.

Metabolic alkalosis can cause mental confusion, seizures, paresthesia, and cramping, and can aggravate cardiac or pulmonary conditions.

RESPIRATORY ACIDOSIS

A high arterial pCO_2 and low pH signify a respiratory acidosis. Acutely, little rise in the HCO_3^- concentration occurs (0.1 mEq/liter per mm Hg). However, if hypercapnia persists, renal H^+ secretion is stimulated and the blood HCO_3^- concentration rises. This process takes several days to complete and is called a *chronic respiratory acidosis.* The increment in HCO_3^- concentration is then about 0.5 mEq/liter for each 1 mm Hg rise in pco_2. Hypercapnia also causes a shift of Cl^- into erythrocytes, a chloriuresis, and hypochloremia.

CO_2 retention is not ascribable to increased CO_2 production but rather to impairment in CO_2 elimination. Common causes include central nervous system depression (drugs, structural lesions), neuromuscular diseases, structural disorders of the thorax (flail chest, pneumothorax), metabolic disturbances (myxedema), airway obstruction, chronic obstructive pulmonary disease, or ventilation/perfusion mismatch.

Symptoms of acute hypercapnia include central nervous system dysfunction (anxiety, headache, confusion, acute psychosis and even coma). Lesser neurologic effects are seen with chronic hypercapnia. Peripheral vasodilation and a propensity to arrhythmias occurs as well.

Treatment of chronic respiratory acidosis rests in improving ventilation. When the pco_2 is normalized, the high HCO_3^- concentration corrects, unless extracellular volume depletion is present, as discussed above.

RESPIRATORY ALKALOSIS

Respiratory acidosis = high arterial pCO_2 and low pH. Respiratory alkalosis = low arterial pCO_2 and high pH.

A low arterial pco_2 and high pH identify a respiratory alkalosis. Only a small decrement in HCO_3^- concentration occurs in acute hypocapnia (0.25 mEq/liter per mm Hg). Over several days, however, a depression of net acid excretion, sometimes with overt bicarbonaturia, is incurred with chronic hypocapnia. The blood HCO_3^- concentration is lowered (0.5 mEq/liter per mm Hg). There is also an associated natriuresis and kaliuresis on a high-salt intake and kaliuresis on a low-salt intake. Lactic acid production is increased acutely by hypocapnia but not chronically.

Important causes of *chronic respiratory alkalosis* include hypoxia of any cause, restrictive lung disease, sepsis, liver disease, salicylate poisoning, structural lesions of the central nervous system, pregnancy, and anxiety.

Symptoms usually relate to the severity of the alkalemia but are seldom clinically important. Acute hypocapnia causes peripheral vasoconstriction and a reduction in cerebral blood flow, which can cause light-headedness, confusion, and occasionally seizures. Treatment is directed at correction of the hypoxia or ventilatory stimulant.

REFERENCES

Reviews

Cogan, M. G., and Rector, F. C., Jr.: Acid-base disorders. *In* Brenner, B. M., Rector, F. C., Jr., eds.: The Kidney, 3rd Edition. W. B. Saunders Co., Philadelphia, 1986.
   This chapter is a comprehensive review of acid-base homeostasis.

Cohen, J. J., and Kassirer, J. P., eds.: Acid-Base. Little, Brown & Company, Boston, 1982.
   This book describes the pathophysiology and clinical manifestations of acid-base derangements.

Diagnosis of Acid-Base Disorders

Narins, R. G., and Emmett, M.: Simple and mixed acid-base disorders: A practical approach. Medicine 59:161–187, 1980.
   This article provides a sound approach to diagnosing acid-base disorders.

Oh, M. S., and Carroll, H. J.: The anion gap. N. Engl. J. Med. 297:814–817, 1977.
The concept and use of the anion gap in diagnosing acid-base disorders is succinctly explained.

Metabolic Acidosis

Arruda, J. A. L., and Kurtzman, N. A.: Mechanisms and classification of deranged distal urinary acidification. Am. J. Physiol. 239:F515–F523, 1980.
A critical and insightful examination of the causes of classic and generalized distal RTA is provided.

Cohen, R. D., and Woods, H. F.: Clinical and Biochemical Aspects of Lactic Acidosis. Blackwell Scientific Publications, Oxford, 1976.
This book provides an authoritative summary of lactic acidosis.

Rector, F. C., Jr., and Cogan, M. G.: The renal acidosis. Hosp. Pract. 15:99–111, 1980.
This article provides an introduction to the diagnosis and pathophysiology of the hyperchloremic metabolic acidoses.

Schambelan, M., Sebastian, A., and Biglieri, E. G.: Prevalence, pathogenesis and functional significance of aldosterone deficiency in hyperkalemic patients with chronic renal insufficiency. Kidney Int. 17:89–101, 1980.
This paper provides one of the most comprehensive reviews of the heterogeneous causes of generalized distal (type IV) RTA.

Metabolic Alkalosis

Cogan, M. G., Liu, F.-Y., Berger, B. E., Sebastian, A., and Rector, F. C., Jr.: Metabolic alkalosis. Med. Clin. N. Am. 67:903–914, 1983.
This article provides a summary of current concepts of the pathophysiology and clinical spectrum of metabolic alkalosis.

Kassirer, J. P., and Schwartz, W. B.: The response of normal man to selective depletion of hydrochloric acid. Factors in the genesis of persistent gastric alkalosis. Am. J. Med. 40:10–18, 1966.
This article is a classic study that exemplifies many aspects of the generation and maintenance of metabolic alkalosis.

Seldin, D. W., and Rector, F. C., Jr.: The generation and maintenance of metabolic alkalosis. Kidney Int. 1:306–321, 1972.
The approach to the pathophysiology, diagnosis, and treatment of the common clinical forms of metabolic alkalosis is presented.

6

Potassium Homeostasis

> **TOTAL BODY POTASSIUM BALANCE**
> Renal Control
> Renal Tubule Transport
> **REGULATION OF POTASSIUM SECRETION**
> Potassium Intake
> Other Factors Affecting Potassium Secretion
> **PATHOGENESIS OF DISTURBANCES IN POTASSIUM HOMEOSTASIS**
> Hypokalemic Disorders
> Hyperkalemic Disorders
> **CLINICAL MANIFESTATIONS OF HYPO- AND HYPERKALEMIA**
> **THERAPY OF HYPO- AND HYPERKALEMIA**

Potassium is the most prevalent cation in body fluids. Total-body potassium content has been estimated at approximately 50 mEq/kg of body weight, or about 3500 mEq. Of total potassium, 98 to 99 per cent is located within cells at an average concentration of 125 mEq/liter. Only about 1 to 2 per cent is in extracellular fluid. Extracellular fluid potassium concentration, however, is closely regulated and seldom varies beyond 3.5 to 4.5 mEq/liter, normally averaging 4 mEq/liter. The marked concentration difference between the potassium concentration in the intracellular fluid (125 mEq/liter) and extracellular fluid (4 mEq/liter) is maintained by the sodium-potassium ATPase pump system which actively transports potassium into and sodium out of all cells in the body.

The importance of maintaining this difference in potassium concentrations across cell membranes stems primarily from the role of potassium in the normal electrical polarization of excitable cells like those in nerve and muscle. When the potassium concentration of the extracellular fluid exceeds 5.5 mEq/liter, *hyperkalemia* is said to exist. Raising the external potassium concentration depolarizes the resting membrane potential and increases cell excitability, eventually leading to cardiac arrest and death. When the potassium concentration of the extracellular fluid is less than 3.5 mEq/liter, *hypokalemia* is said to exist. Lowering the external potassium concentration hyperpolarizes cell membranes and reduces their excitability; when severe this may lead to paralysis, arrhythmias, and death.

Potassium balance is maintained by excreting daily an amount of

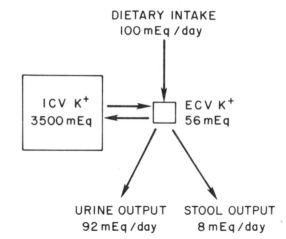

DIETARY INTAKE
100 mEq / day

| ICV K⁺ | | ECV K⁺ |
| 3500 mEq | | 56 mEq |

URINE OUTPUT   **STOOL OUTPUT**
92 mEq / day   8 mEq / day

Figure 6–1. Distribution of potassium in body fluids and maintenance of potassium balance. ICV and ECV, intracellular and extracellular volumes, respectively.

potassium exactly equal to the amount of potassium ingested, normally 100 mEq/day. Potassium excretion can occur through the kidney, gastrointestinal tract, and skin. Normally, however, sweat losses are less than 5 mEq/day and losses in the stools are between 5 and 10 mEq/day; thus the urine is by far the most important route for the excretion of potassium at roughly 92 mEq/day (Fig. 6–1).

Urinary excretion of potassium is normally about 92 mEq/day, or roughly equal to the amount ingested.

TOTAL BODY POTASSIUM BALANCE

Normally plasma potassium concentration is a good index of total body potassium balance. Plasma potassium is usually low during potassium depletion and is increased with potassium excess. During potassium excess and depletion, intracellular potassium acts as a potassium buffer and minimizes alterations in plasma potassium concentration by shifting potassium into or out of cells.

The exchange of potassium between the intracellular and extracellular fluids plays a critical role in the minute-to-minute maintenance of plasma potassium concentration, and is subject to physiologic control by *insulin*, adrenergic nerve activity, and plasma potassium concentration. When dietary potassium is absorbed, the excess is excreted by the kidneys to maintain balance, but the process is slow, requiring several hours. Therefore, initially after potassium ingestion the cellular buffering of excess potassium is essential. Meats and fruits such as oranges, bananas, and especially cantaloupe are very high in potassium. A medium cantaloupe contains approximately 50 mEq of potassium. If this potassium were to be distributed only into extracellular fluid, plasma potassium concentration would increase by a potentially lethal 3.6 mEq/liter. (A 70-kg man has approximately 14 liters of extracellular fluid.) This dangerous increase in plasma potassium is prevented by the rapid entry of potassium into cells. Insulin is believed to play an important physiologic role in the regulation of plasma potassium by activating the sodium-potassium ATPase pump system and promoting the entry of potassium into cells. Thus, with fruit ingestion, insulin secretion promotes the cellular accumulation of both carbohydrates and potassium.

The fasting level of plasma potassium concentration is also partially under the control of insulin. Suppression of basal insulin levels by *somatostatin* results in an increase in plasma potassium concentration of approximately 0.5 mEq/liter. During exercise, potassium is released from muscle, causing acute hyperkalemia. In the postexercise period, potassium moves back into cells by a process dependent on β-adrenergic activity, a process which can be blocked by β-adrenergic antagonists such as *propranolol*. When potassium is lost by vomiting or diarrhea, potassium moves out of cells into the extracellular fluid. Very low plasma concentrations of potassium, on the order of 1 to 2 mM, slow the sodium-potassium ATPase pump system and thus might promote the transfer of potassium from intra- to extracellular fluid.

Renal Control. The kidney plays the major role in control of potassium homeostasis. Potassium in the plasma is freely filtered at the glomerulus. Normally potassium excretion into the urine is between 5 and 15 per cent of the amount of potassium filtered. That excreted potassium is less than filtered potassium demonstrates that there is potassium *reabsorption* along the nephron. Under conditions of excess dietary intake of potassium, however, excreted potassium can exceed filtered potassium as much as twofold, indicating that there is also potassium *secretion* along the nephron. The nephron sites of potassium reabsorption and secretion can be identified by examining the percent of filtered potassium remaining at different sites along the nephron when intake of potassium is normal, low, and high.

The distal nephron is the site of potassium homeostatic control, specifically the collecting tubule.

Under *all* conditions of dietary intake, 85 to 90 per cent of the filtered potassium is reabsorbed in the proximal tubule and the loop of Henle. Urine potassium, however, can be as low as 1 per cent of the amount of potassium filtered at the glomerulus when dietary intake is low or can actually exceed the amount filtered by a factor of two when dietary intake is high. Thus, the distal nephron has the capacity both to secrete and to reabsorb potassium. Since the proximal tubule and the loop of Henle reabsorb potassium at virtually the same rate regardless of dietary potassium intake, these segments are not involved in potassium homeostasis and the rate of potassium excretion is independent of the glomerular filtration rate (GFR). The principal control of potassium homeostasis resides in the distal nephron, and the overall rate of potassium excretion is determined by the rate of potassium secretion in this segment.

Renal Tubule Transport. Tubule transport of potassium can take place by either active or passive transport processes. The principal passive driving force for potassium transport along the nephron is the *transepithelial potential difference (PD)*. The transepithelial PD varies from positive values in the late proximal tubule, favoring potassium reabsorption, to negative values in the late collecting tubule, favoring potassium secretion. At the end of the proximal tubule the PD is lumen-positive 3 mV. The predicted equilibrium luminal potassium concentration for this PD is 3.6 mM, slightly below plasma. Under most conditions of dietary potassium intake the luminal potassium approximates the value predicted for equilibrium with this PD, suggesting that potassium reabsorption in the proximal tubule is passive. In the thick ascending limb of the loop of Henle the transepithelial PD is also lumen-positive by approximately 30 mV. This large lumen-positive PD can account for a great deal of passive cation reabsorption and thus is probably responsible for the large amount of potassium reabsorption in the loop of Henle. Under most circumstances, therefore, potassium reabsorption in the proximal nephron and the loop of Henle can be attributed to passive distribution between tubule fluid and blood in accord with the transepithelial PD.

In contrast to the proximal nephron and the loop of Henle, potassium transport in the distal nephron cannot usually be attributed to passive distribution. Under most circumstances it is necessary to evoke active potassium transport in the collecting tubule. Following dietary potassium deprivation, the entire collecting tubule appears to reabsorb potassium actively; following dietary potassium excess, the entire collecting tubule appears to secrete potassium actively. It is, therefore, the collecting tubule that is capable of responding to dietary intake by either reabsorbing or secreting potassium.

As discussed in Chapter 2, in the collecting tubule there are two cell types concerned with potassium transport: the *principal* (light) cells and the *intercalated* (dark) cells. Both cell types undergo specific morphologic alterations with changes in potassium intake. The principal cells have few mitochondria, a bright appearance, and increase their basolateral infoldings when potassium secretion is stimulated by chronic potassium loading. The principal cells are therefore believed to be responsible for potassium secretion. The intercalated cells have numerous intracellular mitochondria and ribosomes, a dark-to-gray appearance, and increase the density of rod-shaped particles in their luminal membranes when potassium reabsorption is stimulated by dietary potassium restriction. The intercalated cells are therefore believed to be responsible for potassium reabsorption.

Potassium excretion, and thus whole-body potassium homeostasis, is controlled by the collecting tubule, whose principal cells can actively secrete potassium (Fig. 6–2) and whose intercalated cells can actively

In the collecting tubule, intercalated cells are responsible for potassium reabsorption, while principal cells are responsible for its secretion.

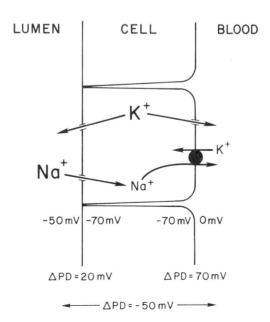

Figure 6–2. Cell model of potassium secretion by collecting duct cells. Potassium secretion appears to occur in principal cells.

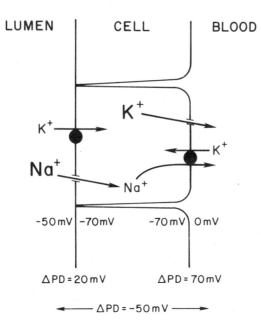

Figure 6–3. Cell model of potassium reabsorption by collecting duct cells. Potassium reabsorption appears to occur in intercalated cells.

reabsorb potassium (Fig. 6–3). It is thought that active potassium reabsorption probably occurs at a relatively constant rate despite modest fluctuations in dietary potassium intake and that the net rate of potassium excretion is governed predominantly by the rate of potassium secretion.

The distal nephron cell responsible for potassium secretion, the principal collecting tubule cell, is depicted in Figure 6–2. The active step in potassium secretion is the sodium-potassium ATPase pump system located in the basolateral or peritubular membrane. The sodium-potassium ATPase pump system creates a high intracellular potassium concentration in these cells, just as it does in every other cell in the body. There are two differences between the principal collecting tubule cell and other body cells: first, the sodium-potassium ATPase pump system is located exclusively on the basolateral cell membrane, just as it is in most renal epithelial cells. Second, and most important for potassium secretion, the passive potassium permeability of the apical membrane is much greater than the passive potassium permeability of the basolateral cell membrane. Thus, although the high intracellular concentration favors passive diffusion of potassium both from cell into lumen and from cell back into interstitial fluid, the greater potassium permeability of the luminal membrane ensures that most potassium diffuses from cell into lumen and that potassium secretion occurs.

There are two steps in active potassium secretion from blood to lumen in the collecting tubule: first, potassium secretion requires active cellular accumulation of potassium at the basolateral cell membrane. Second, potassium secretion involves passive potassium movement from cell to lumen, determined by the electrochemical gradient for potassium across the luminal membrane and the potassium permeability of the luminal membrane. In the distal nephron the chemical concentration gradient across the luminal membrane is the difference between the cell potassium concentration and the potassium concentration in the luminal fluid. The electrical gradient across the luminal membrane is best represented by the transepithelial PD, since the PD between the cell interior and blood is relatively constant. The four primary determinants of potassium movement from cell to lumen are the potassium concentrations in the cell cytoplasm and luminal fluid, the transepithelial PD, and the luminal membrane permeability to potassium. All alterations in potassium secretion can be explained in terms of one or more of these primary determinants.

The four determinants of potassium movement from cell to lumen are:
- *$[K^+]$ in cell cytoplasm*
- *$[K^+]$ in luminal fluid*
- *transepithelial PD*
- *luminal membrane permeability to K^+*

REGULATION OF POTASSIUM SECRETION

Mineralocorticoids such as aldosterone are important regulators of potassium secretion. *Aldosterone* directly influences three of the four primary determinants of potassium secretion: intracellular potassium concentration, potassium permeability of the luminal membrane, and transepithelial PD.

An increase in plasma potassium concentration is a potent and direct stimulus to aldosterone secretion in the *zona glomerulosa* of the adrenal cortex. The mechanism of this effect is probably mediated by the increase in intracellular potassium concentration secondary to the stimulation of the sodium-potassium ATPase pump system by hyperkalemia. Increased intracellular potassium appears to promote aldosterone synthesis by accelerating the conversion of cholesterol to pregnenolone. The mechanism is extremely sensitive. Increases in plasma potassium concentration of 0.1 to 0.2 mEq/liter can induce a significant rise in plasma aldosterone concentrations.

Aldosterone acts on the distal nephron to increase the secretion of potassium and the reabsorption of sodium after a 90-min latent period. Aldosterone enters the cells of the distal nephron by diffusion across the basolateral cell membrane and combines in the cell cytoplasm with a receptor to form an active complex which then enters the cell nucleus. The active complex induces the transcription of both messenger and ribosomal RNA, which leads to increased production of an aldosterone-induced protein. The *induced protein* mediates some of the physiologic effects of the steroid.

Sodium permeability of the luminal cell membrane appears to be increased by the induced protein, either directly or through its stimulation of cellular metabolism. The increase in luminal sodium permeability results in an increased cell sodium concentration which stimulates the activity of the sodium-potassium ATPase pump system. As a consequence, sodium reabsorption and cell potassium concentration are both increased. The stimulation of sodium transport increases the lumen-negative potential difference. Both the increased intracellular potassium concentration and the increased lumen-negative PD are primary determinants for an increase in potassium secretion. In addition, aldosterone appears to directly increase the permeability of the luminal membrane to potassium. This effect occurs immediately and does not appear to require the induced protein. The increase in luminal membrane potassium permeability means that for any concentration gradient of potassium between cell and luminal fluid there is a greater potassium movement.

Aldosterone directly increases the permeability of the luminal membrane to potassium.

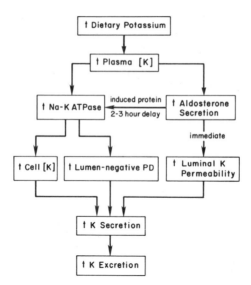

Figure 6–4. Regulation of renal potassium excretion by dietary potassium intake.

Potassium Intake. The main determinant of potassium secretion is potassium intake. Potassium secretion increases when dietary potassium is high and decreases when it is low. The effect of dietary potassium on potassium secretion appears to be mediated by changes in the plasma potassium concentration. Plasma potassium influences potassium secretion in two ways: first, there is an effect of plasma potassium concentration directly on the sodium-potassium ATPase pump system in the basolateral cell membrane. High plasma potassium stimulates sodium-potassium ATPase and low plasma potassium inhibits the enzyme. Alterations of the sodium-potassium ATPase pump system alter the potassium concentration inside the cells of the distal nephron. Second, increased dietary potassium stimulates the secretion of aldosterone, which will further enhance potassium secretion as described above. Figure 6–4 shows how increased plasma potassium concentration influences the sodium-potassium ATPase pump system and aldosterone secretion during an increase in dietary potassium uptake. A similar diagram, but with arrows reversed, could be drawn for a potassium-deficient diet. In addition, during potassium-deficient dietary intake there appears to be an increase in the potassium reabsorptive mechanism probably by an active potassium uptake step in the luminal membrane of the intercalated cells (Fig. 6–3).

Other Factors Affecting Potassium Secretion. In addition to the influence of mineralocorticoids and dietary intake on potassium secretion and the control of potassium homeostasis, potassium secretion is also influenced by other factors.

Distal Nephron Flow Rate. Potassium is almost completely reabsorbed in the proximal nephron and the loop of Henle, causing the potassium concentration entering the distal nephron to be low, perhaps as low as 1 mEq/liter. As the tubule fluid passes the potassium secretory cells, potassium enters the fluid and raises the potassium concentration while reducing the concentration difference for potassium between the tubule cells and the tubule fluid. The decrease in the potassium concentration gradient will retard potassium flux from cell to tubule

In the proximal nephron and loop of Henle, nearly complete potassium reabsorption occurs.

fluid. This decrease is dependent on the tubule flow rate adjacent to the secretory site. If the flow rate is slow, a large increment in tubule fluid potassium concentration is produced by potassium movement from cell to lumen. As a result, at slow flow rates potassium secretion is minimal. If tubule fluid rate is very fast, then the increase in tubule fluid potassium concentration produced by potassium movement from cell to lumen is minimized because secreted potassium is washed downstream. As a result, potassium secretion is stimulated, increasing flux rates. At extremely fast distal tubule fluid flow rates there is no longer an influence of flow rate on potassium secretion. This plateau in potassium secretion at very high flow rates is caused by reaching the minimal tubule fluid potassium concentrations and the maximal potassium concentration difference between cell and tubule fluid. Faster flow rates cannot increase this gradient further.

In Figure 6–5 the relationship between distal tubule fluid flow rate and distal potassium secretion at different levels of potassium intake is described. The shaded area represents the normal range of distal nephron flow rate. At both high and normal potassium intakes there is a marked and direct relationship between flow rate and potassium secretion. The slope of the relationship is determined by the intracellular potassium concentration and the potassium permeability of the luminal membrane which is under the control of aldosterone. The low potassium condition appears to be insensitive to flow rate, probably because the potassium permeability of the luminal membrane in the absence of mineralocorticoid is essentially zero. In addition, there is probably some stimulation of potassium reabsorption on a low potassium diet.

The most common means of increasing the flow rate in the distal nephron, and thus increasing potassium secretion, is by using diuretics. Proximal and loop diuretics inhibit sodium, chloride, and water reabsorption, thereby increasing the delivery of fluid to the distal nephron potassium secretory site. In addition to the flow effect in the distal nephron, proximal diuretics can also increase net potassium excretion by inhibiting proximal and loop potassium reabsorption. In general, potassium-sparing diuretics, which impair sodium and potassium transport in the collecting tubule, shift the flow rate vs. potassium secretion curves (Fig. 6–5) downward toward a level appropriate for a lesser potassium intake.

Diuretic administration is the most common means of increasing distal nephron flow rate and thus potassium secretion.

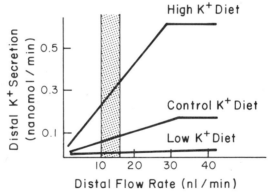

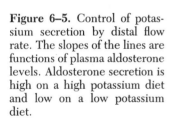

Figure 6–5. Control of potassium secretion by distal flow rate. The slopes of the lines are functions of plasma aldosterone levels. Aldosterone secretion is high on a high potassium diet and low on a low potassium diet.

Distal Nephron Sodium Delivery. There is a direct relationship between sodium delivery to the distal nephron and potassium secretion. Potassium secretion is reduced when sodium delivery is reduced and increased when sodium delivery is increased. It is, however, difficult to separate the effects of sodium delivery alone from the effects of distal tubule flow rate and transepithelial PD. Usually, conditions that increase distal tubule sodium delivery, such as diuretic administration, also increase distal tubule flow rate. For the most part, effects of sodium delivery can be attributed to effects of flow and PD. There is, however, a definite requirement for some sodium (approximately 15 mEq/liter) in the distal tubule fluid because of the exchange nature of the sodium-potassium ATPase pump system. But since the rate of sodium reabsorption with chloride or bicarbonate exceeds the rate of potassium secretion by a factor of at least ten, and normally enough sodium to prime the sodium-potassium ATPase pump is present, sodium delivery is not rate-limiting.

Distal Nephron Anion Permeability. The transepithelial PD in the distal nephron is lumen-negative as a result of active sodium reabsorption. Potassium secretion is favored by a lumen-negative PD. The more negative the PD, the greater the potassium secretion. Clearly, factors which influence the active rate of sodium reabsorption will alter the PD and thus influence potassium secretion. In addition, there is an indirect effect of the anion permeability on the magnitude of the PD. At any given rate of active sodium transport the PD will be more lumen-negative when more poorly permeable anions are present in the distal tubule fluid. The effect of anion permeability on the magnitude of the transepithelial PD is due to the mechanism by which the PD is generated. Active transport of the cation Na^+ will generate a lumen-negative PD because the sodium potassium ATPase pump system will move positively charged ions from lumen to blood. The lumen-negative PD then drives the luminal anion from tubule fluid to blood, thus shunting the lumen-negative PD. The more easily the anion can permeate the membrane, the greater the shunting of the lumen-negative PD. In the distal nephron, Cl^- is more permeable than HCO_3^- or $SO_4^=$. When Cl^- is the major anion in the distal tubule fluid, the PD is less lumen-negative than when HCO_3^- or $SO_4^=$ are the distal anions. The less permeable anions enhance the lumen-negative PD and favor K^+ secretion. Similarly, an increase in the Cl^- content or in the Cl^- permeability of the distal nephron will tend to reduce the transepithelial PD and favor K^+ retention.

Systemic Acid-Base Status. Acid-base disturbances alter potassium excretion. At any given plasma potassium concentration alkalosis increases and acute acidosis decreases potassium secretion. The mechanism of this effect on potassium excretion appears to be through alterations in intracellular potassium concentration (Fig. 6–6). Acidosis causes potassium to leave the cell, and alkalosis causes potassium to enter the cell. The increase in cell potassium concentration in alkalosis and the decrease in cell potassium concentration in acidosis results in parallel changes in potassium secretion.

The potassium retention that occurs during the first 24 hours of acidosis is invariably overridden by other factors (Fig. 6–6). In acidosis there is a depression of sodium, chloride, and water reabsorption in

The more negative the transepithelial PD in the distal nephron, the greater the potassium secretion.

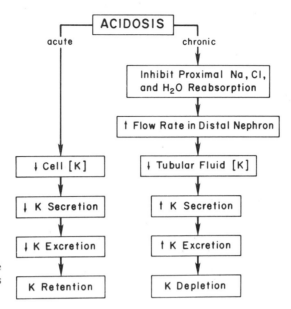

Figure 6–6. Effects of acute and chronic metabolic acidosis on potassium balance.

the proximal tubule. As a result the amount of fluid reaching the distal nephron is increased. Increased distal flow rate keeps the potassium concentration in the distal tubule flow low, maintaining a high potassium concentration difference between cell and tubule fluid and thereby enhancing potassium secretion. Thus, in chronic acidosis potassium secretion is actually enhanced despite the fact that intracellular potassium concentration is depressed. In summary, the direct effect of acidosis on intracellular potassium concentration is overridden by the secondary effects of acidosis on distal nephron flow rate. Ultimately, then, all acid-base disturbances generate enhanced potassium excretion and potassium depletion.

All acid-base disturbances generate enhanced potassium excretion and depletion.

PATHOGENESIS OF DISTURBANCES IN POTASSIUM HOMEOSTASIS

Hypokalemic Disorders (Table 6–1). Plasma potassium concentration tends to parallel body stores of potassium. A fall in plasma potassium concentration from 4.0 to 3.0 mEq/liter requires the loss of approximately 3 per cent (100 mEq) of total body potassium; a fall to 2.0 mEq/liter requires the loss of about 10 per cent. This relationship between plasma concentration and total body stores can be obscured by factors that specifically influence the distribution of potassium between cellular and extracellular compartments. Acute alkalosis and acidosis are particularly important in this respect. An increase in blood pH of 0.1 unit will lower plasma potassium by 0.5 to 1.0 mEq/liter, while a 0.1 unit fall in pH will raise plasma potassium by 0.5 to 1.0 mEq/liter. In diabetic ketoacidosis the combination of acidosis, hyperosmolality, and insulin lack will result in hyperkalemia, despite total body potassium deficits. In contrast, glucose and insulin can lower potassium concentration even in the face of excess total body potassium.

Table 6–1. CAUSES OF POTASSIUM DEFICIENCY AND HYPOKALEMIA

Inadequate intake
Gastrointestinal loss (diarrhea, laxatives, vomiting)
Renal loss
    Mineralocorticoid excess
        Primary hyperaldosteronism
            Conn's syndrome
            Bilateral adrenal hyperplasia
        Nonaldosterone mineralocorticoid
            Cushing's syndrome, adrenogenital syndrome
        Secondary hyperaldosteronism
            Renin-secreting tumor
            Renovascular hypertension
            Accelerated hypertension
    Decreased salt reabsorption proximal to the collecting tubule
        Diuretics
        Osmotic diuretics
        Bartter's syndrome
        Magnesium deficiency
    Distal delivery of a nonreabsorbable anion
        Penicillins
        Ketoacidosis
        Metabolic alkalosis (vomiting, sodium bicarbonate ingestion)
        Proximal and distal renal tubular acidosis
        Acetazolamide
    Acid-base changes
        Metabolic alkalosis
        Chronic metabolic acidosis

These factors which can influence the distribution of potassium must be considered in the evaluation of patients for evidence of potassium deficiency.

Causes of potassium deficiency can be grouped into three separate categories: (1) decreased intake, (2) gastrointestinal losses, and (3) renal losses. As will be discussed, there is some overlap among these groups.

Inadequate dietary potassium intake is rarely a cause of hypokalemia.

Inadequate Dietary Intake. This is an unusual cause of hypokalemia unless patients go extended lengths of time without potassium ingestion. This is in marked contrast to sodium. If a person stops eating sodium, urinary and fecal losses will go almost to zero. However, on a zero potassium diet, urinary losses will never fall below 5 mEq/day, and stool losses never below 5 to 10 mEq/day. Thus a person ingesting less than 10 to 15 mEq/day of potassium will eventually become potassium-depleted and hypokalemic.

Gastrointestinal Loss. The two most common causes of hypokalemia are vomiting and diarrhea. It is, however, an oversimplification to group these entities under gastrointestinal losses. The potassium concentration of gastric, pancreatic, or small intestinal secretions rarely exceeds 10 mEq/liter. Thus to accrue a deficit of 200 mEq would require 20 liters of vomiting. Vomiting is in fact associated with much greater degrees of potassium depletion, but the mechanism is not gastric loss of potassium. Vomiting leads to volume depletion, high aldosterone levels, and severe metabolic alkalosis; the combination of increased delivery of bicarbonate to the distal nephron and high aldosterone levels produces intense renal potassium wasting. In addition, as is discussed below, alkalosis leads to redistribution of potassium into cells, further worsening the hypokalemia in an already potassium-depleted patient.

Diarrhea, on the other hand, can cause true fecal potassium wasting. However, the acidosis frequently seen in diarrhea can lead to some degree of renal potassium wasting and an inappropriately elevated urinary potassium. In addition, the acidosis will cause potassium to be redistributed extracellularly, leading to a degree of hypokalemia that does not accurately reflect the severity of potassium depletion.

Renal Loss. Most causes of hypokalemia involve renal potassium wastage. A normally functioning kidney in the presence of hypokalemia will maintain urinary potassium excretion less than 20 to 30 mEq/day. Urinary potassium in excess of this in the presence of hypokalemia indicates renal potassium wasting. Most forms of hypokalemia caused by renal potassium loss can be explained by one or more of the four abnormalities already discussed: (1) ↑ mineralocorticoids; (2) ↑ distal delivery of sodium and volume; (3) ↑ distal delivery of nonreabsorbable anions, and (4) acid-base alterations.

When dietary sodium chloride intake is varied, the effects of mineralocorticoids and distal delivery counterbalance each other such that under normal circumstances potassium excretion is independent of volume status. Decreases in extracellular volume increase aldosterone secretion while decreasing distal delivery. Increases in extracellular volume status suppress aldosterone but increase distal delivery. Disruption of this balance explains many of the renal forms of hypokalemia.

Under normal circumstances potassium excretion is independent of volume status.

Mineralocorticoid Excess. In pathologically significant forms of mineralocorticoid excess, the increased mineralocorticoid activity cannot be attributed to decreased extracellular fluid volume. These conditions lead to salt retention, expansion of extracellular volume, and a high incidence of hypertension, but not edema. A so-called "escape" will occur before sufficient salt is retained for edema formation. In these conditions, normal or increased extracellular fluid volume leads to normal or increased distal delivery in the presence of high mineralocorticoid levels, and thus there is renal potassium wasting.

Mineralocorticoid excess can result from a number of conditions. Primary aldosteronism refers to conditions where the cause of excess aldosterone secretion is a primary adrenal disease. In its most common form, this condition is caused by a benign tumor of the zona glomerulosa and is referred to as Conn's syndrome. Renin levels are low, aldosterone levels are high, hypertension is uniformly present (with the exception of a few rare case reports), and hypokalemic alkalosis is common. Removal of the tumor corrects all of the abnormalities. Less commonly, primary aldosteronism is caused by bilateral hyperplasia of the adrenal zona glomerulosa. Hypokalemia secondary to mineralocorticoid excess is also a feature of diffuse bilateral adrenocortical hyperplasia (Cushing's syndrome). In this instance, the potassium wasting is a result of the mineralocorticoid effects of the naturally occurring glucocorticoids. In other instances, i.e., adrenogenital syndromes, the potassium wasting is caused by excessive production of the mineralocorticoid desoxycorticosterone (DOC). In both Cushing's and adrenogenital syndromes plasma renin activity and aldosterone levels are low.

Hyperaldosteronism can also be caused by excess renin secretion which is inappropriate to the volume status. This occurs with renin-producing tumors, renovascular hypertension, accelerated hypertension, and occasionally secondary to birth control pills. In this situation, increased aldosterone levels are secondary. Patients with these disorders are hypertensive and hypokalemic with elevated plasma aldosterone and renin levels.

In all of the above causes of mineralocorticoid excess, *hypertension* and *alkalosis* are common in addition to the hypokalemia. Plasma renin activity and aldosterone levels are frequently helpful in distinguishing these entities.

Decreased Salt Reabsorption. Inhibition of salt reabsorption proximal to the collecting tubule increases distal delivery and leads to small degrees of volume depletion which will secondarily elevate plasma renin activity and aldosterone levels. The combination of increased aldosterone levels and increased distal delivery leads to increased renal potassium wasting and hypokalemia. This group of disorders is different from the previous group in that elevated aldosterone levels are appropriate for the mildly decreased extracellular fluid volume, and hypertension is usually not a feature.

Diuretic ingestion is the most common cause of renal potassium loss.

The most common cause of renal potassium wasting is diuretic ingestion. As is obvious from the above discussion, any diuretic that acts proximal to the cortical collecting tubule will increase renal potassium excretion. This includes diuretics that act in the proximal tubule, such as acetazolamide; diuretics that act in the loop of Henle, such as furosemide and ethacrynic acid; and diuretics that work in the early distal tubule, such as the thiazides. In addition, diuretics that work in the loop of Henle may inhibit potassium reabsorption in this segment.

Osmotic diuresis will also lead to potassium wasting by this mechanism. Osmotic diuresis occurs in poorly controlled diabetes mellitus when serum glucose rises to higher levels than the proximal tubule can absorb. In addition, osmotic diuretics, such as mannitol or urea, are used therapeutically in some conditions.

Bartter's syndrome is a rare condition in which there appears to be a primary defect in salt reabsorption by the loop of Henle. This leads to chronic increases in distal delivery and a chronic state of mild volume contraction. Patients are hypokalemic, with very high renin and aldosterone levels. Blood pressure is normal or low.

Magnesium deficiency may mimic Bartter's syndrome by causing hyperreninemic hyperaldosteronism and potassium wasting in the absence of hypertension.

All penicillins are nonreabsorbable anions.

Increased Distal Delivery of Nonreabsorbable Anions. In certain conditions, sodium is delivered distally with a nonreabsorbable anion. As discussed, this will increase the lumen-negative PD and lead to increased potassium wasting. All penicillins are nonreabsorbable anions; however only a few of these are given in sufficient quantities to lead to significant potassium wasting. Carbenicillin and ticarcillin are examples of these. Ketoacids will act as nonreabsorbable anions in patients with ketoacidosis caused by diabetes, alcoholism, or starvation. In addition, HCO_3^- can function as a nonreabsorbable anion if it is delivered to the distal nephron in greater amounts than can be reabsorbed. This occurs during the active phase of vomiting, acute respiratory alkalosis, proximal renal tubular acidosis, and acetazolamide administration.

Acid-Base Changes. As discussed, all chronic acid-base disorders can lead to some degree of potassium wasting. However, metabolic alkalosis, both acute and chronic, clearly leads to the most marked degree of hypokalemia because of the increased collecting tubule cell potassium concentration, distal delivery of HCO_3^- (behaving as a nonreabsorbable anion), and redistribution of potassium into cells. Metabolic acidosis may also lead to mild degrees of potassium depletion as a result of decreased proximal salt absorption, but frequently extracellular redistribution of potassium prevents hypokalemia.

Diagnostic Approaches. The cause of hypokalemia is usually obvious in edematous or hypertensive patients known to be taking diuretics. However, in other patients the cause can be enigmatic. Blood pressure, urine electrolytes, and plasma renin activity all provide useful diagnostic information. Hypokalemic hypertensive patients having normal urine sodium, potassium, and chloride values reflecting normal dietary intake can be considered to have renal potassium wasting. If the plasma renin activity is depressed, then the patient must be evaluated for some form of mineralocorticoid excess by measurement of adrenal steroid levels. If, on the other hand, the plasma renin activity is high, then unreported diuretic ingestion or some form of secondary hyperaldosteronism must be considered. In hypertensive patients with low urine potassium and sodium levels, the hypokalemia is usually caused by earlier diuretic ingestion, dietary restriction, or fecal loss through diarrhea or laxatives.

In hypokalemic, alkalotic, nonhypertensive patients the associated mild-to-moderate volume depletion results in elevations of plasma renin activity and aldosterone levels; therefore these values usually have little diagnostic importance. The urine electrolytes and pH, however, are particularly useful. If the urine sodium and potassium are high, the chloride low, and the urine pH high (7.0 or greater) the patient is either actively vomiting (either acknowledged or surreptitious) or ingesting sodium bicarbonate. Once the patient stops vomiting and the generation of new bicarbonate in plasma ceases, the urine sodium, potassium, and chloride will all be low and the urine pH will be 6.5 or less. If the urine electrolytes and pH are normal the most likely possibility is surreptitious diuretic ingestion, with or without associated magnesium deficiency. This should be evaluated by screening the urine for the presence of diuretics. Only after this possibility is excluded should one seriously consider the possibility of Bartter's syndrome.

To make a diagnosis of Bartter's syndrome, one must first rule out active vomiting, $NaHCO_3$ ingestion, and diuretic ingestion, all of which may be surreptitious.

In hypokalemic, nonhypertensive patients with mild-to-moderate hyperchloremic acidosis, the differential diagnosis includes chronic diarrhea, laxative abuse, and some form of proximal or distal renal tubular acidosis. This differentiation is complicated by the fact that the steatorrhea, vitamin D deficiency, and secondary hyperparathyroidism found in chronic "sprue-like" states can cause renal tubular acidosis. Differentiation of these disorders is discussed in Chapter 5, but should include measurements for phenolphthalein, magnesium, or other laxative agents in stools and urine.

Hyperkalemic Disorders (Table 6–2). As described in the begin-

Table 6–2. CAUSES OF HYPERKALEMIA

Excessive intake
Decreased renal excretion
    Renal insufficiency
        Acute renal failure
        Chronic renal failure
    Decreased mineralocorticoid activity
        Addison's disease
        Adrenal biosynthetic defects
        Hyporeninemic hypoaldosteronism
    Distal tubular defect
        Intrinsic renal disease
        Amiloride, spironolactone, triamterene
Cellular redistribution
    Cell death
    Acidosis
    Hyperosmolality
    Succinylcholine
    Hyperkalemic periodic paralysis

ning of this chapter, the body has a marked ability to protect against hyperkalemia. This includes regulatory mechanisms that excrete excess potassium quickly and redistribute excess potassium into cells until it is excreted. All causes of hyperkalemia involve abnormalities in this regulation.

In assessing a patient with a high measured serum potassium concentration, it is important to remember that not all of these patients have *"true" hyperkalemia.* Because cell potassium concentrations are large and serum potassium concentrations are small, small leaks of potassium out of cells can have large effects on measured serum potassium. Normally when blood is allowed to clot before centrifugation, enough potassium is released from platelets to raise serum potassium concentration by approximately 0.5 mEq/liter. This is accounted for in the limits of normal. However, excessive errors can occur in the presence of marked thrombocytosis, marked leukocytosis, or hemolysis on obtaining the blood sample. These conditions are referred to as *"pseudohyperkalemia."*

Excessive Dietary Intake. Because of the regulatory defense mechanisms, excessive intake is an unusual cause of hyperkalemia. In the presence of normal renal and adrenal function it is difficult to ingest enough potassium to become hyperkalemic. It is even more difficult to do this on a chronic basis because of *potassium adaptation.*

Decreased Renal Excretion. Decreased renal excretion of potassium can result from one or more of three abnormalities: (1) ↓ distal delivery of salt and water; (2) ↓ mineralocorticoids; and (3) abnormal cortical collecting tubule function.

Renal Insufficiency. As discussed, most of filtered potassium is reabsorbed before the distal tubule. Potassium excretion is then determined by the rate at which potassium is secreted in the distal nephron. The acute decreases in GFR that occur in acute renal failure would therefore not be expected to have a marked effect on potassium excretion. Acute decreases in GFR may, however, lead to marked decreases in distal delivery of salt and water which may secondarily decrease distal potassium secretion. Thus, when acute renal failure is oliguric, hyperkalemia is a frequent problem. When acute renal failure is nonoliguric, however, distal delivery is usually sufficient and hyperkalemia is unusual.

Chronic renal failure is more complicated than acute renal failure. In addition to the decreased GFR and secondary decrease in distal delivery, there is *nephron dropout* and fewer collecting tubules to secrete potassium. However, this is counterbalanced by a poorly understood potassium adaptation, in which the remaining nephrons develop an increased ability to excrete potassium. This adaptation can be prevented by decreasing dietary potassium in proportion to the decrease in renal function. In addition, these patients possess two other defenses against hyperkalemia. First, in response to a potassium load, potassium redistributes into cells faster than normal. Second, there is a markedly increased rate of potassium excretion in the stools. Thus, although patients with chronic renal failure do not excrete a potassium load as fast as normal patients, hyperkalemia is unusual until chronic renal failure has progressed to GFRs of less than 5 ml/min. The occurrence of hyperkalemia with a GFR of 10 to 50 ml/min should raise the question of decreased aldosterone levels or a specific lesion of the cortical collecting tubule (see below).

Decreased Mineralocorticoid Activity. Decreased aldosterone levels lead to decreased potassium excretion and hyperkalemia, and can occur alone or in combination with decreased cortisol levels. Addison's disease is the deficiency of aldosterone and cortisol resulting from destruction of the adrenal glands. Rarely, selective hypoaldosteronism may occur as a result of a primary adrenal defect, but much more commonly is a secondary response to impaired renin secretion (hyporeninemic hypoaldosteronism).

Hyporeninemic hypoaldosteronism occurs in patients with chronic renal insufficiency. It is especially common in patients with diabetic nephropathy or interstitial renal disease. Renin and aldosterone levels are both low and the primary defect is decreased renin production by the kidney. When patients with moderate degrees of renal insufficiency develop hyperkalemia, this is a frequent cause. Evaluating aldosterone secretory rates in these patients is complicated by the direct effects of hyperkalemia on the adrenal glands. Commonly, the aldosterone levels appear normal while the patient is hyperkalemic, but will fall to abnormally low levels when serum potassium is reduced to normal.

Distal Tubule Defect. Certain renal diseases can affect the distal nephron specifically and lead to hypokalemia in the presence of only mild decreases in GFR and normal or elevated aldosterone levels. In most cases this is caused by a defect in potassium secretion. In a few patients, a high chloride permeability in the collecting tubule decreases the transepithelial PD, thus inhibiting potassium secretion and leading to hyperkalemia. In addition, certain diuretics impair the ability of the cortical collecting tubule to secrete potassium. *Amiloride* and *triamterene* inhibit sodium transport, which makes the transepithelial PD less negative and secondarily inhibits potassium secretion. *Spironolactone* competes with aldosterone for its receptor and thus blocks the mineralocorticoid effect. Although these diuretics are useful in patients with a hypokalemic tendency, they weaken an important defense mechanism

Oliguria (scanty urine output) in acute renal failure is likely to cause hyperkalemia. In nonoliguric acute renal failure, hyperkalemia is unusual.

Certain diuretics such as amiloride, triamterene, and spironolactone weaken hyperkalemia defense mechanisms and should be avoided in patients predisposed to hyperkalemia.

against hyperkalemia and should therefore be avoided in patients with other defects predisposing to hyperkalemia (i.e., diabetes mellitus, chronic renal insufficiency).

Cellular Redistribution. Cellular redistribution is more important as a cause of hyperkalemia than of hypokalemia. Hyperkalemia that results from redistribution of potassium out of cells is caused primarily by tissue damage. This damage can be caused by rhabdomyolysis, trauma, burns, tumor lysis (following treatment), or massive intravascular coagulation.

Sudden increases in plasma osmolality will cause potassium to move out of cells. This most frequently occurs in diabetic patients when their blood glucose rises. In addition, certain anesthetics such as succinylcholine act by depolarizing cell membranes. This causes potassium to leave cells. Acidosis, either metabolic or respiratory, will cause potassium to move out of cells and lead to hyperkalemia.

Last, *periodic paralysis* also occurs in a hyperkalemic form. Patients are well except for brief episodes when potassium redistributes out of their cells and paralysis and hyperkalemia develop.

CLINICAL MANIFESTATIONS OF HYPOKALEMIA AND HYPERKALEMIA

Hypokalemia (Table 6–3). The most important clinical manifestation of hypokalemia occurs in the neuromuscular system where low serum potassium leads to cell hyperpolarization, thus impeding impulse conduction and muscle contraction. Typically, a *flaccid paralysis* develops in the hands and feet and moves proximally to eventually include the trunk and respiratory muscles. Death may occur from respiratory insufficiency.

Table 6–3. CONSEQUENCES OF HYPOKALEMIA

Neuromuscular
  Flaccid paralysis
  Myopathy $+/-$ Rhabdomyolysis
  CNS changes
  Paralytic ileus
Cardiac
  Tachyarrhythmias
  Impaired myocardial function
Vascular
  Decreased response to catecholamines, postural hypotension
  Impaired exercise-induced vasodilation
Renal
  Decreased glomerular filtration rate
  Impaired urine concentrating ability, polyuria
  Sodium retention
  Metabolic alkalosis
Endocrine
  Impaired insulin release
  Glucose intolerance
  Decreased glycogen synthesis
  Decreased aldosterone production, increased sweat sodium

A *myopathy* may also occur which in its most severe form can lead to frank rhabdomyolysis and renal failure. Potassium deficiency prevents exercise-induced vasodilation and consequently is an important factor in the rhabdomyolysis, heat injury, and renal failure occurring secondary to strenuous exercise.

Hypokalemic damage to the neuromuscular system can range from postural hypotension to fatal paralysis of respiratory muscles.

Hypokalemia can also lead to CNS changes including confusion and affective disorders, smooth muscle dysfunction with paralytic ileus, and mild autonomic insufficiency with postural hypotension.

Cardiac complications of hypokalemia are also important. The typical electrocardiogram (ECG) change is ST depression, T wave flattening, and an increased U wave. This change, often misread as a widened QT, is nonspecific, often absent, and of little clinical use. It is well known that hypokalemic patients on cardiac glycosides have an increased incidence of premature ventricular contractions and supraventricular and ventricular tachyarrhythmias. There is now an increasing awareness that hypokalemia can predispose to these arrhythmias even in patients not on these drugs.

Hypokalemia also affects the kidney. Its most pronounced effect is a concentrating defect resulting from a decrease in the medullary gradient. In extreme cases, it may produce mild *nephrogenic diabetes insipidus*. It can also cause sodium retention, occasionally to the point of edema. Hypokalemia stimulates renal ammoniagenesis and thus contributes to the development of metabolic alkalosis.

Because insulin release is regulated partially by serum K, hypokalemia can lead to glucose intolerance.

Hyperkalemia. All of the clinically important manifestations of hyperkalemia occur in excitable tissue. This is because the electrical potential across the cell membranes is partly determined by the ratio of intracellular to extracellular potassium. Hyperkalemia thus leads to depolarization, which causes a resetting of the threshold for initiating the action potential and a *depolarization block*. Conduction velocity is markedly slowed.

In hyperkalemia, excitable tissue is the site of all clinically important manifestations.

The heart is certainly the most sensitive to these changes and the effects are easily observable in the ECG (Fig. 6–7). The first sign in the ECG is a peaking of the T wave. Then the QRS and PR widen. Eventually, the P wave will disappear and the QRS and T wave may together form what appears as a *sine wave*. This is a harbinger of ventricular fibrillation and death. The correlation of ECG changes with serum potassium depends on the rapidity of onset of the hyperkalemia. Generally with acute onset of hyperkalemia, ECG changes appear at a serum K of 6 to 7 mEq/liter. However, with chronic hyperkalemia, the ECG may remain normal up until serum potassium of 8 to 9 mEq/liter. *Treatment of hyperkalemia is based more on the ECG than on the value of the serum potassium.* All patients should have serum potassium corrected, but those with ECG changes should be treated quickly. Patients with QRS widening or sine waves should be treated as emergencies.

Neuromuscular manifestations may also occur in hyperkalemia, but are less common. Paresthesia in the arms and legs is followed by a symmetrical flaccid paralysis beginning in the hands and feet and moving proximally. Trunk, head, and respiratory muscles are spared.

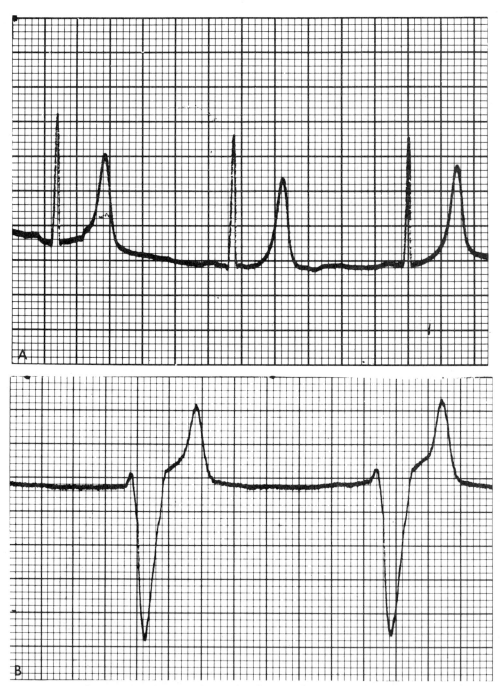

Figure 6–7. Characteristic electrocardiographic changes during hyperkalemia. (A) Symmetrical peaked T waves and normal P-R interval and QRS duration in a patient with a serum potassium level of 7.1 mEq/liter. (B) More serious cardiotoxicity in a patient with a serum potassium level of 8.6 mEq/liter. In addition to peaked T waves, the P waves are absent, indicating atrial standstill, and the QRS duration is markedly prolonged.

THERAPY OF HYPOKALEMIA AND HYPERKALEMIA

Acute Hypokalemia. As with all disorders, the best therapy for acute hypokalemia is to treat the cause. In addition, potassium should be given to the patient in order to replace the potassium deficit and correct the serum potassium. Generally, if correction of hypokalemia is not urgent, oral therapy is indicated. If intravenous therapy is indicated, potassium should be administered at a rate not to exceed 10 mEq/hr, unless treatment is urgent. Generally the potassium concentration in the IV fluid should be less than 40 to 80 mEq/liter. When potassium is given intravenously it is usually in the form of KCl.

The choice of an oral preparation of potassium is difficult. The most commonly used is liquid KCl, which unfortunately has a very unpleasant taste. $KHCO_3$ or potassium citrate have a much more pleasant taste but these will cause the patient's bicarbonate to rise, leading to bicarbonaturia. The bicarbonate will then carry the potassium out in the urine. KCl has also been administered as an enteric coated pill which dissolves in the stomach. This unfortunately led to gastric ulceration and is no longer available. Presently a pill is available that contains KCl in a matrix (Ilo-K). This appears not to cause ulceration.

Chronic Hypokalemia. When the cause of potassium wasting cannot be corrected, chronic treatment is indicated. This can be in the form of chronic oral KCl treatment; however, as already mentioned, the taste is unpleasant. If renal potassium wasting is a problem, renal potassium excretion can be decreased with potassium-sparing diuretics (spironolactone, amiloride, triamterene), but they remove an important defense against hyperkalemia and should never be given in conjunction with oral KCl. The advantage of oral KCl alone is that renal defenses against hyperkalemia remain intact in the event a patient is overdosed.

Acute Hyperkalemia (Table 6–4). When hyperkalemia is acute, the treatment depends on the electrocardiogram. If the ECG shows widening of the QRS, treatment should be started with intravenous calcium. This reverses the effect of hyperkalemia on the heart and works within 20 to 30 sec of administration. In addition, treatment to move potassium into cells should be given with intravenous $NaHCO_3$ or glucose plus insulin. This treatment can be given alone if the ECG shows peaked T waves. Last, potassium needs to be removed from the body. If the patient has good renal function, diuretics that increase distal delivery can be used. Frequently, however, these patients do not have good renal function and a potassium-binding resin should be administered orally or as an enema. In the intestinal tract potassium

In acute hypokalemia, potassium replacement is given orally or intravenously. In chronic hypokalemia, either potassium is replaced orally or potassium-sparing diuretics are given, but never both.

In acute hyperkalemia, calcium or $NaHCO_3$, or both should be given intravenously. In chronic hyperkalemia either diuretics are given or dialysis is required.

Table 6–4. ACUTE TREATMENT OF HYPERKALEMIA

Antagonize cellular effect
    $CaCl_2$
Shift K into cells
    $NaHCO_3$
    Insulin + glucose
Remove K^+ from the body
    Resins
    Dialysis
    Diuretics

binds to the resin and subsequently is excreted in the stool. An alternative treatment is dialysis (hemodialysis or peritoneal dialysis) with potassium-free solutions which will effectively and rapidly remove potassium from the body.

Chronic Hyperkalemia. If patients have good kidney function, potassium excretion can frequently be increased with diuretics (furosemide or thiazides) or mineralocorticoid (in mineralocorticoid deficiency states). If kidney function is poor, dialysis may be necessary.

REFERENCES

Wright, F. S., and Giebisch, G.: Renal potassium transport: Contributions of individual nephron segments and populations. Am. J. Physiol. 4:F515–F527, 1978.

Gennari, F. J., and Cohen, J. J.: Role of the kidney in potassium homeostasis: Lessons from acid-base disturbances. Kidney Int. 8:1–5, 1975.

Giebisch, G., Malnic, G., and Berliner, R. W.: Renal transport and control of potassium excretion. *In* Brenner, B. M., and Rector, F. C., Jr., eds.: The Kidney, 3rd Edition. W. B. Saunders Co., Philadelphia, 1986.

Sebastian, A., Hernandez, R., and Schambelan, M.: Disorders of renal handling of potassium. *In* Brenner, B. M., and Rector, F. C., Jr., eds.: The Kidney, 3rd Edition. W. B. Saunders Co., Philadelphia, 1986.

These are excellent and comprehensive reviews of current understanding of renal potassium handling in health and disease.

7

Calcium, Phosphorus, and Magnesium

NORMAL METABOLISM

In a normal adult of constant weight, the kidneys excrete each day as much calcium, phosphorus, and magnesium as the intestinal tract absorbs; and if dietary intake of any mineral declines substantially, intestinal absorption and renal tubule reabsorption both become efficient enough to conserve endogenous stores. During growth and pregnancy, intestinal absorption rises above urinary losses so these three materials can accumulate in newly formed bone and soft tissues, whereas bone disease or loss of lean body mass increases urinary mineral loss without a balanced increase of intestinal absorption. Intestinal absorption and renal excretion are linked mainly by *parathyroid hormone (PTH)* and the active form of vitamin D, *1,25(OH)$_2$D$_3$*, which control mineral transfer across intestinal and renal tubule epithelia, and are themselves regulated by serum levels of calcium and phosphorus.

Intestinal Absorption. Net intestinal absorption, the absolute difference between dietary intake and fecal excretion, rises with intake, but differently for each mineral (Fig. 7–1). Phosphorus and magnesium absorption rise linearly with intake, and fall to zero when intake is very low. Calcium absorption rises more slowly; in the range of 10 to 20

The absolute difference between dietary intake and fecal excretion is termed "net intestinal absorption."

153

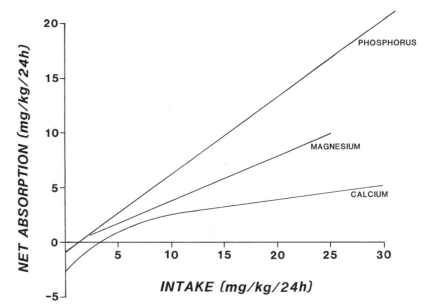

Figure 7–1. Effects of dietary intake on net intestinal absorption of calcium, phosphorus, and magnesium.

mg/kg of intake usually encountered, it is virtually constant. Below 10 mg/kg/day of intake, absorption falls steeply and becomes negative, as fecal losses exceed dietary supply because of calcium secretion by intestine and in pancreatic, biliary, and salivary juices.

In jejunum, phosphorus absorption is very extensive (Fig. 7–2).

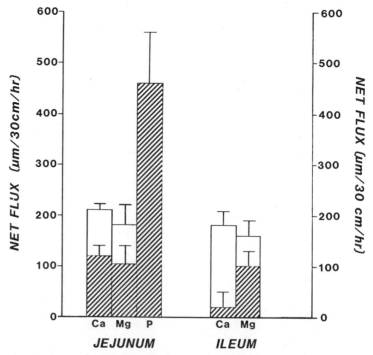

Figure 7–2. Segmental transport of calcium, magnesium, and phosphorus in human jejunum and ileum.

Calcium and magnesium also are both absorbed; their absorption rates increase when dietary intake is reduced (clear areas of bars), but absorptive fluxes remain below that of phosphate. In ileum, calcium absorption is very low when dietary intake is normal, but rises greatly during low calcium diet. Magnesium handling by ileum is like that of jejunum, except that absorption is less markedly reduced by high calcium diet. In jejunum, calcium and magnesium transport processes are saturable, whereas phosphate absorption is not.

Virtually every segment of intestine from the rat has been studied in vitro to determine transport rates of calcium and phosphate in the absence of electrical or chemical gradients, conditions under which net movement across the tissue usually reflects active transport. Net calcium absorption occurs mainly across duodenum, cecum, and colon; phosphorus is absorbed mainly by jejunum, and by duodenum when $1,25(OH)_2D_3$ is available. $1,25(OH)_2D_3$ stimulates almost all segments to absorb both minerals.

Net calcium absorption occurs across the duodenum, cecum, and colon; phosphorus is absorbed by jejunum and duodenum; magnesium is insufficiently studied to predict its site(s) of absorption.

If one combines these in vitro data with human studies, the overall impression is that $1,25(OH)_2D_3$ can stimulate calcium transport from mucosa to serosa along the whole length of the bowel, so that local transport rates increase and the total surface over which absorption increases becomes very large. Phosphate absorption, however, is mainly by jejunum and duodenum, even when $1,25(OH)_2D_3$ is plentiful. In vitro studies of magnesium fluxes are not available.

Cellular Mechanisms of Calcium Transport. The net movement of calcium is the difference between mucosal to serosal (Jms) and serosal to mucosal (Jsm) fluxes. In duodenum and colon, studied in vitro, Jms exceeds Jsm and is saturable, whereas Jsm rises linearly with calcium concentration over a wide range and does not saturate. A reasonable interpretation is that Jms occurs by active transcellular transport, in which brush border, cytoplasm, and basolateral membranes are traversed, whereas Jsm is mainly paracellular.

Calcium entry across the brush border could occur passively, because cytosolic ionic calcium concentrations are in the micromolar range and the cell interior is negatively charged compared with extracellular fluid. Subsequent extrusion at the basolateral membrane, however, must proceed against both chemical and electrical driving forces, and is therefore usually viewed as an active step that depends on a local energy source, perhaps arising from the hydrolysis of *adenosine triphosphate (ATP)*.

In experiments with intact cells and membrane vesicles, calcium movement seems passive across the brush border and active at the basolateral membrane. There is an ATPase in basolateral membranes that has a high calcium affinity. Altogether the evidence favors extrusion of calcium by a high affinity calcium-ATPase, which could be offset by a sodium-calcium exchange mechanism. $1,25(OH)_2D_3$ has no influence on basolateral vesicle transport. It does, however, increase passive calcium uptake by brush border vesicles in rabbit and chicken, and may therefore stimulate calcium transport by increasing access of the ion into the cytosol and therefore to basolateral active transport sites.

The opposite flux, Jsm, probably is paracellular, occurring through the channels between cells. Such a flux could arise from diffusion of calcium through water in paracellular channels, and also from convective movement of calcium in the direction of whatever net water movement might occur. Diffusive and convective transport are both unsaturable, as Jsm is, and would also vary in a predictable way with the transmembrane PD. In colon and cecum, voltage dependence of Jsm suggests diffusive or convective transport. Neutral sugars such as mannitol move across intestinal tissue, and mannitol Jsm is parallel to that of calcium; since mannitol does not enter cells appreciably, the similarity of the two fluxes supports paracellular calcium movement.

Phosphate transport in the cell is strongly dependent on sodium transport.

Cellular Mechanisms of Phosphate Transport. Especially in jejunum, Jms greatly exceeds Jsm for phosphate, indicating the effects of active transport mechanisms. Most attention has been given to the absorptive flux, which seems to reflect secondary active transport coupled to sodium transport. Entry of phosphate across the brush border is strongly opposed by the transmembrane PD, since phosphate is an anion and the cell interior is electrically negative compared with extracellular fluid. Extrusion of phosphate at the basolateral membrane, however, would be favored by the PD. In duodenum, and less so in ileum, phosphate influx across the mucosal surface consists of a saturable component that is sodium-dependent and an unsaturable component that does not depend upon sodium availability. In studies of pH dependence and effects of membrane potential, the sodium-dependent component seemed to involve neutral sodium phosphate movement. $1,25(OH)_2D_3$ stimulates sodium-dependent phosphate uptake by brush border vesicles, by increasing the Vmax of the entry step. Jsm for phosphate has not been studied in detail. It is unknown whether it is saturable, sodium-dependent, and parallel to the flux of a paracellular marker like mannitol.

$1,25(OH)_2D_3$ is the major regulator of intestinal Ca, P and Mg absorption.

Regulation of $1,25(OH)_2D_3$. This hormone is the major regulator of intestinal calcium, phosphate, and magnesium absorption, and variation of its availability to intestinal cells is critical in modulating mineral balance. The hormone is manufactured in mitochondria of proximal tubule and pars recta cells, by 1-α-hydroxylation of $25(OH)D_3$, the latter synthesized in liver cells by 25-hydroxylation of vitamin D_3. Serum $25(OH)D_3$ levels can alter $1,25(OH)_2D_3$ production by changing substrate availability, but this occurs mainly, if not exclusively, in states of D_3 deficiency or pathologic excess. Apart from states of vitamin D deficiency or intoxication, $25(OH)D_3$ levels are constant and do not increase in response to growth, low calcium or phosphorus diet, and pregnancy, even though $1,25(OH)_2D_3$ levels rise greatly. This suggests that normal physiological regulation depends more upon variation of renal 1-α-hydroxylation than hepatic hydroxylation at the 25 position.

Effects of PTH. The biologically active fragment of native PTH, consisting of the first 34 amino acids beginning at the amino-terminal end, can increase serum $1,25(OH)_2D_3$ levels in humans and rats. In normal and hypoparathyroid people, PTH raises $1,25(OH)_2D_3$ levels. It also lowers serum phosphorus and raises calcium levels, however, so it is hard to distinguish effects of altered serum ion concentration from a direct hormone action on renal tubule cells. Some experiments have, however, dissociated effects of PTH upon $1,25(OH)_2D_3$ from changes in serum calcium and phosphorus. PTH can stimulate in vitro conversion of $^3H-24(OH)D_3$ into $^3H-1,25(OH)_2D_3$ by tubule fragments from kidneys of vitamin D-deficient chicks. These facts are evidence for a direct action of PTH on $1,25(OH)_2D_3$ production.

Effects of Calcium and Phosphate. Dietary phosphate deficiency raises serum calcium and lowers serum PTH, yet greatly raises serum $1,25(OH)_2D_3$ level. An increase in $1,25(OH)_2D_3$ also occurs when thyroparathyroidectomized (TPTX) rats are phosphate-depleted. Low calcium diet can raise serum $1,25(OH)_2D_3$ in normal and TPTX rats, even when serum phosphate is allowed to rise. But the effects of low calcium diet are much reduced in TPTX rats, whereas effects of low phosphate diet are not, suggesting that part of the calcium effects are mediated by PTH. Overall, low serum phosphate and calcium both appear to stimulate $1,25(OH)_2D_3$ production, and the direct effects of phosphate exceed those of calcium; however, low serum calcium also raises PTH, so in intact animals reduced intakes or serum levels of either raise $1,25(OH)_2D_3$ production markedly.

Low serum levels of phosphate or calcium seem to stimulate production of $1,25(OH)_2D_3$.

Circulating Forms of $1,25(OH)_2D_3$. About 99 percent of both $25(OH)D_3$ and $1,25(OH)_2D_3$ in serum is bound to a protein whose serum concentration varies. Binding complicates the interpretation of serum $1,25(OH)_2D_3$ measurements because total steroid concentrations may not reflect hormone available to tissues but simply variations in the binding protein. Tissues that respond to $1,25(OH)_2D_3$, intestine, bone and, perhaps, kidney, have receptors for the hormone whose affinities may affect extraction from blood. Since it is technically very difficult to measure even total circulating $1,25(OH)_2D_3$, and few laboratories can measure the protein (bound and unbound fractions are not yet reliably measurable), mechanisms of hormone regulation based upon contemporary studies of total circulating $1,25(OH)_2D_3$ are provisional.

Regulation of PTH. The main determinant of peripheral PTH activity appears to be PTH secretion by the parathyroid glands, even though the secreted hormone is rapidly degraded into fragments that circulate in blood. Like many peptide hormones PTH exerts its tissue effects mainly by stimulating cellular production of *cyclic adenosine monophosphate (cAMP)* after attaching to high affinity, specific receptors on kidney and bone cells.

Secretion. The parathyroid glands contain some PTH, stored in granules. Preformed PTH is released in response to a fall in the extracellular ionic calcium concentration $[Ca^{++}]$. A sustained reduction of $[Ca^{++}]$ activates the synthesis of new messenger RNA for PTH, and subsequently an increased synthesis of the protein. If parathyroid glands, in vivo, are subjected to chronic reduction of $[Ca^{++}]$, the cells increase their rate of division, and the glands enlarge because of hyperplasia. Altogether, the glands respond in such a way that immediate and long-term increases in PTH secretion accompany reduced serum $[Ca^{++}]$.

Parathyroid glands increase PTH synthesis and release in response to a decline in extracellular ionic calcium concentration.

PTH secretion also responds to extracellular ionic magnesium concentration $[Mg^{++}]$. Reduced $[Mg^{++}]$ increases PTH secretion even if $[Ca^{++}]$ is normal; but when $[Mg^{++}]$ falls below 0.8 mg/100 ml, PTH secretion falls even if $[Ca^{++}]$ is low. PTH secretion is less responsive to altered $[Mg^{++}]$ than $[Ca^{++}]$ as judged by in vitro studies of hormone release. Catecholamines may influence PTH secretion, but their effects are not fully established. $1,25(OH)_2D_3$ appears to suppress PTH secretion.

Blood Ionized Calcium. The critical role of $[Ca^{++}]$ in PTH secretion may well be a biological adaptation to the extreme importance of this ion in general. A very stable value of [Ca^{++}], 1.15 mM/liter, is needed for proper function of the mammalian nervous system, cardiac conduction pathways, and both cardiac and skeletal muscle. [Ca^{++}] is also critical in determining the calcium-phosphate ion product of the extracellular fluid in equilibrium with bone mineral.

Blood calcium participates in multiple equilibria that influence [Ca^{++}] by direct chemical interaction. *Serum albumin*, an anionic protein, normally binds about 50 percent of calcium; the percentage falls with lowered pH. Calcium also forms complexes, mainly with CO_3^- and phosphate, that account for 10 percent of total calcium. The remainder is free ionized calcium. Calcium complexes and [Ca^{++}] are ultrafilterable. Because [Ca^{++}] varies inversely with blood pH and serum phosphorus concentration, chronic phosphate retention, as in renal failure, can cause secondary parathyroid hyperplasia, whereas a sudden increase of blood pH, as in respiratory alkalosis, can provoke hypocalcemic tetany.

Peripheral Metabolism. Liver, kidney, and bone can cleave native 1–84 PTH into an active fragment incorporating the first 34 amino acids (amino terminal fragment) and an inactive 35–84 fragment *(carboxy terminus fragment)*; all three molecules may contribute to PTH levels as measured by immunoassay. The native hormone is biologically active and has a very brief life in the circulation of about 15 min. The 1–34 fragment, which has all of the activity of the native hormone, is taken up by bone and kidney and rapidly metabolized; it has a half life of 100 min. The 35–84 fragment is biologically inactive. It is filtered by the renal glomeruli and excreted, has a half life of many hours, and therefore is the major form of PTH in blood. Peripheral PTH metabolism may not regulate delivery of active PTH to bone and kidney because native hormone and the 1–34 fragment have equal biological activity and metabolic conversion of native hormone to fragments cannot affect total circulating PTH activity. However, the rapid clearance of biologically active PTH makes serum PTH activity very responsive to rapid changes in PTH secretion.

Measurement of PTH and cAMP. Fragments complicate the interpretation of PTH measurements. Radioimmunoassay depends upon attachment of antibody to circulating hormone fragments, and depending on the antibody, an assay may be most sensitive to 35–84 fragments ("C-terminal" assays), 1–34 fragments ("N-terminal" assays), or to some midportion of the molecule. Because they have a long life in the circulation, 35–84 fragments attain a serum concentration that tends to reflect average secretory rates over a period of many hours, whereas native hormone and 1–34 levels closely parallel rapid variations of secretory rate. C-terminal assays are therefore best at detecting chronic PTH oversecretion, as in primary hyperparathyroidism, and N-terminal assays are best for short-term physiological studies. In chronic renal failure, 35–84 fragments accumulate because they normally are excreted by glomerular filtration. Serum PTH values become very elevated if a C-terminal immunoassay is used, even though the serum level of active PTH molecules (native hormone + 1–34 fragments) may be increased modestly.

Urine cAMP is frequently measured as an index of tissue PTH effects, which cannot be easily derived from serum PTH level alone.

In general, urine cAMP is elevated in states of chronic PTH excess. The measurement is more valuable if the contribution of filtered cAMP is subtracted using measured serum cAMP values and glomerular filtration rate.

Renal Handling of Calcium, Magnesium, and Phosphate. *Urinary Excretion.* As net intestinal absorption of the three minerals rises, their urine excretion rates also rise, but at differing rates (Fig. 7–3). Phosphate excretion rises along the line of identity. Calcium excretion rises very slowly, so as net absorption exceeds 2 mg/kg/day, positive net balance can increase progressively. However, because it is closely regulated, calcium absorption tends to remain between 1 and 3 mg/kg/day (Fig. 7–1) even as calcium intake varies from 5 to 15 mg/kg/day, so calcium balance generally is near zero. Magnesium excretion is like that of calcium, and since absorption ranges between 1 and 4 mg/kg/day (Fig. 7–1) on most diets, balance is near zero.

Glomerular Filtration. All three materials are less than completely filtered, as judged by comparing serum concentrations to concentrations in either an ultrafiltrate produced by an artificial membrane, in vitro, or fluid aspirated by micropuncture from Bowman's space. Because albumin-bound calcium is not filtered only 65 to 70 percent of total calcium is ultrafilterable in humans and in the rat. The percent of ultrafilterable phosphate is 85 to 88 and is about 80 percent for magnesium. The importance of incomplete filtration is that the filtered load of an ion must be calculated using measured values for the ultrafilterable fraction. There are no known physiological or regulatory functions that depend upon variation of the ultrafilterable fraction.

Only 65 to 70 percent of total calcium, but 80 percent of magnesium and 85 to 88 percent of phosphate is filterable.

Overall Tubule Reabsorption. After filtration, the three ions are reabsorbed at different rates along the tubule (Fig. 7–4). In PTH-replete, euvolemic rats, 65 to 70 percent of calcium and magnesium leave the proximal convoluted tubule compared with only 32 percent of the phosphate. By the early distal convoluted tubule, only 10 to 15 percent of calcium and magnesium remain unreabsorbed, presumably due to further reabsorption by pars recta and the loop of Henle, but most of the phosphate that leaves the proximal convoluted tubule enters the distal convoluted tubule. Almost all of the remaining calcium

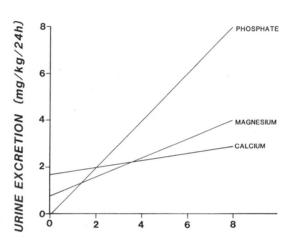

Figure 7–3. Relationship between urinary excretion and intestinal net absorption of calcium, phosphate, and magnesium.

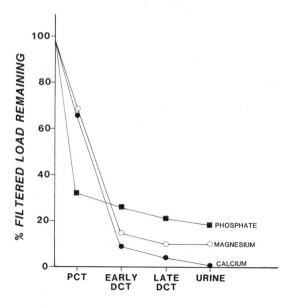

Figure 7–4. Fractional reabsorption of filtered calcium, phosphate, and magnesium along the nephron as disclosed by micropuncture. PCT, proximal convoluted tubules; DCT, distal convoluted tubules.

is reabsorbed between the distal convoluted tubule and urine, whereas most of the magnesium and phosphate that leave the distal convoluted tubule enter the urine. As a result, about 10 percent of filtered magnesium and 20 percent of filtered phosphorus are excreted in the urine, compared to 1 percent or less of filtered calcium.

PTH and ECF volume are the major regulators of overall renal handling of Ca, P and Mg.

Regulation of Reabsorption. PTH and ECF volume are the two major regulators. Thyroparathyroidectomy (TPTX) has little effect upon the amount of filtered calcium that reaches the late distal convoluted tubule, but fractional excretion of calcium in the urine rises from less than 1 to 6 percent. This implies that PTH must exert a critical calcium-conserving effect on nephron segments between the distal convoluted tubule and urine. Overall excretion of filtered magnesium is barely altered by TPTX despite increased magnesium delivery to and out of the distal convoluted tubule. TPTX greatly reduces phosphate delivery out of the proximal convoluted tubule and distal convoluted tubule, and fractional excretion of phosphate falls markedly.

ECF volume expansion in the intact rat increases excretion of all three minerals. But even though delivery of calcium to the distal convoluted tubule is increased, the fraction of filtered load reaching the late distal convoluted tubule is about the same as in TPTX or intact rats. Thus, either volume expansion reduces calcium reabsorption by late nephron segments, or delivery out of the late distal convoluted tubule is elevated only in deep cortical nephrons whose distal convoluted tubule cannot be micropunctured and these nephrons account for increased calcium excretion. Volume expansion increases delivery of magnesium to the early distal convoluted tubule; delivery to the late distal convoluted tubule has not been measured. Phosphate delivery out of the proximal convoluted tubule and distal convoluted tubule is increased by ECF expansion, and phosphaturia is marked since late nephron segments exhibit little phosphate reabsorption.

Segmental Calcium and Phosphate Reabsorption. Transport by tubule segments, in vitro, has been extensively studied for calcium and phosphate, but magnesium studies are very limited because the only available radioisotope has a very short half-life. In the proximal convoluted tubule (Fig. 7–5), phosphate flux greatly exceeds that of calcium, a difference consistent with micropuncture data showing greater fractional reabsorption of phosphate than calcium (Fig. 7–4). Phosphate transport is not altered by PTH, in vitro, even though micropuncture results have documented increased delivery out of the proximal convoluted tubule in response to PTH administration. This discrepancy has not yet been explained. In the pars recta (Fig. 7–5), calcium reabsorption exceeds that of phosphate. PTH reduces phosphate reabsorption but its effects on calcium transport are unknown. No net phosphate movement occurs across thin or thick segments of the loop of Henle and permeability to passive movement also is low. This is consistent with micropuncture data, since the decrease in fractional delivery of phosphate between the proximal convoluted tubule and the early distal convoluted tubule could easily reflect the effects of the pars recta. There also is no active calcium movement across the thin limbs of Henle's loop, and passive permeability is as low for calcium as it is for phosphate. The thick ascending limb of Henle's loop, however, offers a great contrast because calcium is

There is no active calcium movement across the thin limbs of Henle's loop, but extensive reabsorption in the thick ascending limb.

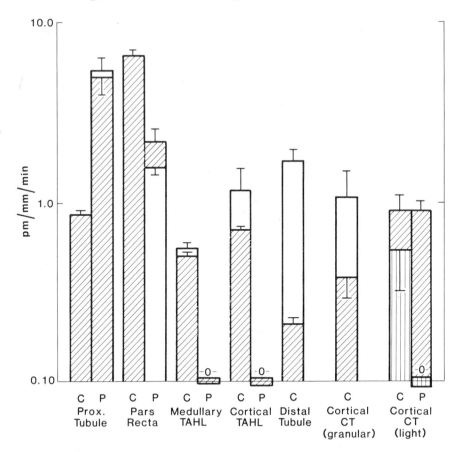

Figure 7–5. Segmental reabsorption of calcium and phosphorus along the nephron, as studied by in vitro tubule microperfusion techniques. Clear areas show transport rates in the presence of PTH; diagonal shaded bars show results in tubule segments that have not been stimulated by PTH. Vertical shading on the last group of bars indicates the effects of vasopressin.

extensively reabsorbed. Reabsorption by the thick ascending limb of Henle's loop could well explain why calcium fractional delivery to the distal convoluted tubule is low compared with phosphate. In the absence of PTH, medullary and cortical thick ascending limbs have similar net calcium fluxes; PTH increases that of the cortical, but not the medullary, segment.

In contrast to other areas of the nephron, the thick ascending limb of Henle's loop normally maintains its lumen positive by 15 to 25 mV with respect to the basolateral surface. Such a transmembrane potential favors passive calcium movement from lumen to blood.

The late distal convoluted tubule and granular portion of the cortical collecting tubule both reabsorb calcium and respond to PTH. These segments may account for the steep, PTH-dependent, increase in fractional reabsorption that occurs between the last distal convoluted tubule portion accessible to micropuncture and the final urine. No phosphate studies have been done for the distal convoluted tubule. The cortical collecting tubule may reabsorb phosphate but probably not calcium.

Segmental Magnesium Reabsorption. In vitro fluxes across tubule segments are not yet available, but in vivo microperfusion studies have documented that in the proximal tubule, along the length of Henle's loop, and in the distal convoluted tubule, absolute absorptive fluxes rise progressively with increasing perfusate $[Mg^{++}]$ and without clear saturation. In the loop of Henle, reabsorption is reduced by hypermagnesemia, but stimulated by PTH. PTH and hypermagnesemia do not alter reabsorption by in vivo perfused proximal or distal convoluted tubules. These findings cannot be compared directly with in vitro perfusion, but they suggest a major role of loop segments in magnesium regulation, under control of PTH. This is compatible with the large fall in fractional magnesium delivery between the proximal and early distal convoluted tubule as revealed by micropuncture.

Segmental Effects of PTH. PTH is thought to affect transport by stimulating production of cAMP, and cAMP production by tubule segments in response to PTH does correlate well with PTH effects on transport. PTH causes marked cAMP and transport responses in the late distal convoluted tubule, a moderate response in the proximal convoluted tubule and cortical thick ascending limb, and slight response in pars recta and cortical collecting tubule; no cAMP response occurs in the medullary thick ascending limb or the early distal convoluted tubule. In the medullary segment, the lack of transport and cAMP response correspond well, as do the positive responses of cAMP and transport in other segments.

Effects of Drugs and Hormones Other Than PTH. The nature of calcium and phosphate transport has been explored using responses to drugs and hormones apart from PTH. *Ouabain*, an inhibitor of Na-K ATPase, inhibits calcium and phosphate transport of the proximal convoluted tubule; in pars recta, calcium transport is unaffected by ouabain but phosphate transport is inhibited. Ouabain does not reduce calcium reabsorption by the medullary thick ascending limb. These results are comparable to intestinal studies in which calcium transport by duodenum and jejunum have been unaffected by ouabain, and data showing dependence of phosphate uptake by brush border vesicles upon sodium. Furosemide inhibits calcium reabsorption by the medullary, but not the cortical thick ascending limb, a difference that is not yet explained. cAMP stimulates calcium reabsorption by the medullary and cortical segments, but PTH acts only on the cortical limb. This suggests that the medullary thick ascending limb has no PTH receptors but does possess the cellular machinery to respond to peptide hormones. The medullary segment does produce cAMP in response to calcitonin, and calcitonin increases calcium reabsorption in that segment, but not in the cortical thick ascending limb.

Bone Handling of Calcium, Magnesium, and Phosphate. Bone mineral is the major reservoir of calcium in the body, in the form of *calcium phosphate crystals*. The crystals are described as a form of apatite, but their exact crystalline structure is not certain. Each crystal is much longer than it is wide, and the crystals cover the surface of a collagen substrate in an orderly pattern. Some magnesium and carbonate are included in the solid phase. The calcium-phosphorus ratio of bone is about 4:5.

Calcium in bone mineral is crystalline calcium phosphate, produced by osteoblasts (bone cells).

Mineralization. The normal blood product of calcium $[Ca^{++}]$ and phosphate $[P^=]$ ions exceeds the solubility limit for bone mineral, so crystals could form and grow spontaneously, but the orderly production of crystal is governed by bone cells called *osteoblasts*. These cells appear to accumulate calcium and phosphorus, releasing the two minerals, possibly as a solid phase, at specific sites in the cartilage of growing animals, and along the collagenous bone matrix in both growing and adult animals whose bones are undergoing normal turnover (*remodeling*).

Mineralization seems to depend upon both an adequate $[Ca^{++}][P^=]$ product and the presence of vitamin D. It seems likely that $25(OH)D_3$ or $1,25(OH)_2D_3$ can permit bone to mineralize, so both must be deficient to interfere with mineralization.

Turnover. Mineralized bone is broken down by multinucleated bone cells called *osteoclasts*, and in the adult breakdown is balanced exactly by remineralization elsewhere. This process permits constant remodeling of the bone. PTH promotes demineralization; when present in excess, it causes net loss of mineral. Osteoclasts will not attack *unmineralized osteoid*, bone matrix that does not contain crystals. Therefore, if mineralization is prevented by vitamin D deficiency or a low blood $[Ca^{++}][P^=]$ product, osteoid that is newly produced during turnover will accumulate. The unmineralized osteoid is deposited on bone surfaces as an initial step in remineralization, and if it does not mineralize, the bone becomes inactive, with low turnover.

Regulation of Bone Mineral. Total bone mineral is the net result of differences between production and degradation, and to a great extent these two processes are linked either intrinsically or by hormones other than PTH and vitamin D. Normal growth of bone can occur in PTH deficiency. Excess PTH can cause demineralization, insufficient vitamin D can prevent mineralization, and, possibly, excessive vitamin D can promote demineralization, but no known variations of these two hormones above or below their normal values can cause bone to increase its mineral stores.

Regulation of Blood Mineral Concentrations. *Effects of Transport Rates.* The transport activities of intestinal and renal epithelia, the net uptake rate of bone and, in the case of phosphorus and magnesium, the body cell mass, are the major factors that determine blood mineral concentrations. Their effects can be given quantitative expression simply by assuming that all three minerals are neither created nor destroyed anywhere within the organism.

[i]: Blood concentration of ionized Ca, P, or Mg

[F]: Blood concentration of ultrafilterable Ca, P, or Mg

γ: $[i] \div [F]$ (this symbol is needed in the derivation)

r: Fractional reabsorption of filtered Ca, P, or Mg by renal tubules

α: Fraction of dietary Ca, P, or Mg absorbed by the intestine

D: Dietary supply of Ca, P, or Mg

β: Fraction of D retained in the body for Ca, P, or Mg

U: Urine concentration of Ca, P, or Mg

V: Urine flow rate

g: Glomerular filtration rate (GFR)

We may express the definition of r as:

$$UV = g[F](1\text{-}r) \tag{1}$$

This is true, because r is the fraction of filtered mineral (g[F]) not excreted, and we have assumed exact conservation of total mineral. Also by assuming conservation:

$$D(\alpha\text{-}\beta) = UV \tag{2}$$

In other words, mineral absorbed ($D\alpha$) and not retained ($D\beta$) is excreted in the urine.

Combining Equations 1 and 2:

$$D(\alpha\text{-}\beta) = g[F](1\text{-}r) \tag{3}$$

By rearrangement:

$$[F] = \frac{D(\alpha\text{-}\beta)}{g} \times \frac{1}{1\text{-}r} \tag{4}$$

Using γ:

$$[i] = \frac{D(\alpha\text{-}\beta)}{g} \times \frac{\gamma}{1\text{-}r} \tag{5}$$

Equation 5 indicates that ionized blood concentration must vary linearly and directly with $D\alpha$ and γ, linearly and negatively with β, and inversely with g and the term (1-r). It also shows that the ratio of urine excretion, $D(\alpha\text{-}\beta)$ to GFR, in units of mass/time $\div$ volume/time, yields the concentration term mass $\div$ volume, which is scaled by the unitless value (1/1-r) to give [i]. Since [i] is similar for all mammals, excretion rates for minerals are best expressed per unit GFR to allow comparisons between individuals of different size.

Hormone Integration. A system of regulation emerges if the effects of D, α, β, g, and r upon [i] implied by Eq. 5 are added to effects of PTH upon r and β; of PTH, [P$^=$], and [Ca^{++}] upon $1,25(OH)_2D_3$; of $1,25(OH)_2D_3$ upon α; and of ionized calcium upon PTH (Fig. 7–6).

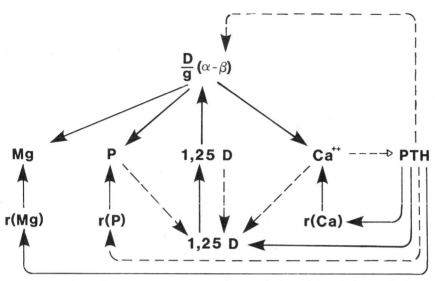

Figure 7–6. Overall diagram showing regulation of mineral metabolism. D, dietary supply of calcium, phosphorus, or magnesium; g, glomerular filtration rate; α, fractional absorption of mineral by intestine; β, fraction of dietary supply retained by the body cell mass and skeleton; 1,25D, $1,25(OH)_2D_3$; PTH, parathyroid hormone; fractional reabsorption is indicated throughout by lower case r; Mg, magnesium; P, phosphorus; Ca, calcium; Ca^{++}, ionized calcium; continuous lines indicate upregulation; dotted lines indicate downregulation.

Solid lines indicate direct, dotted lines negative or inverse effects. Certain minor effects, or effects observed only during disease are not shown; e.g., of [Mg] on PTH, of elevated Ca^{++} to reduce g, of low values of $[P^=] \times [Ca^{++}]$ to reduce bone mineralization and, therefore, β. The diagram also cannot reveal the quantitative differences between effects of altered α, β or D, and g or r upon serum values. The first three exert linear effects, whereas effects of g and r are hyperbolic. For example, variation of r over the physiological range for calcium, of 95 to 99 percent, causes a change of 1/(1-r) from 20 to 100.

Normal Values. The blood value for $[Ca^{++}]$ is very close to 1.15 mM/liter despite wide variation of D. The range for g in normal people is about 100 to 200 liters/day, and over this range Eq. 5 shows that r need vary only slightly to keep $[Ca^{++}]$ content (Fig. 7–7) yet accommodate to values of calcium excretion between 40 mg/day, the lowest extreme of normal, and 300 mg/day, the upper limit. Calcium excretion rates above 300 mg/day raise urine supersaturation with respect to calcium oxalate and calcium phosphate enough that the risk of calcium renal stones becomes appreciable, so r(Ca) cannot be permitted to fall much below 95 percent even at a g of 100 liters/day. Serum total phosphorus is about 1.1 mM, but more variable than calcium (1 to 1.5 mM); values for ultrafilterable phosphate as a percent of the total are about 80 percent. Urine excretion rates are much larger, 500 to 1000 mg/day, and if 1.15 is used as a value for $[P^=]$, values of r are much lower at all values of g. Values for total serum magnesium are about 0.82 mM and daily excretion about 100 mg (4.1 mM), so values of r are a bit lower than for calcium; for example, 95.6 percent at 100 and 97 percent at 200 liters/day of g. For simplicity, magnesium is not shown in Figure 7–7.

Normal calcium excretion rates range from 40 to 300 mg/day.

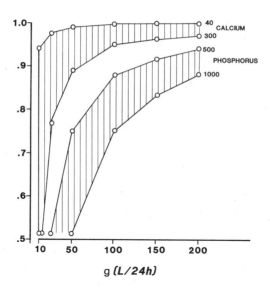

Figure 7–7. Relationship between fractional reabsorption, glomerular filtration rate, and urinary excretion for calcium and phosphorus necessary to maintain the blood ionized calcium at 1.15 mm/liter and the blood phosphorus level at 1 mm/liter. As glomerular filtration rates (g) fall, fractional reabsorption (r) must fall in a curvilinear and accelerating manner at any given value of urine excretion, in order to maintain constant blood values. The shaded zone spans the region between the lower and upper limits of the normal range for calcium or phosphorus loss in the urine.

Response to Normal Variations. The intestinal tract, kidneys, bone, and parathyroid glands can be viewed as parallel processors of the blood (Fig. 7–8) in that each receives the same arterial blood as inflow and alters its composition as it traverses the capillaries, producing a venous effluent that differs from the arterial blood and varies the total blood composition. This new composition becomes the inflow to each organ. In Figure 7–8, values of Q, blood flow, and the venous (v) minus arterial (a) concentration are shown for calcium, phosphorus, PTH, and $1,25(OH)_2D_3$; arterial blood values for all four are displayed at the top of the figure. The horizontal axes of all the graphs depict time, from onset of a change to the point at which a new equilibrium is reached. Vertical axes have normal set-points (N) and an o-point placed in proper relation to N.

Low Calcium Diet. D (Ca) is suddenly reduced, with no other changes, to virtually 0. Delivery, Q(v-a), of calcium into the portal veins (Fig. 7–9) falls below 0 because calcium secretion is no longer balanced by epithelial absorption and blood $[Ca^{++}]$ falls. PTH production and blood [PTH] rise; low $[Ca^{++}]$ and high [PTH] raise $1,25(OH)_2D_3$ production and blood levels. PTH also causes bone mineral dissolution that increases bone Q(v-a) for calcium and phosphorus and PTH raises r(Ca) and lowers r(P). $1,25(OH)_2D_3$ raises gut absorption of Ca and P; since D(Ca) is zero, the only effect is to reabsorb secreted calcium so Q(v-a)Ca becomes 0; αP rises. Blood $[Ca^{++}]$ is returned toward normal by increased r(Ca), bone Q(v-a), and a less negative gut value of Q(V-a)Ca. Blood $[P^=]$ is under two opposing influences, reduced r(P) and increased bone and gut delivery, and is depicted as stable. $[Ca^{++}]$ rises, and [PTH], $[1,25(OH)_2D_3]$, and bone Q(v-a) fall so that by equilibrium there is slight hypocalcemia; however, secondary hyperparathyroidism, elevated $[1,25(OH)_2D_3]$, reduced r(P), increased r(Ca), elevated urine phosphorus, very low urine calcium, and chronic depletion of bone mineral all remain. Calcium and phosphorus balance may be detectably negative, reflecting bone demineralization. A lesser degree of calcium restriction, one that permits values of intestinal Q(v-a)Ca at equilibrium tᴏ be positive, will give the same

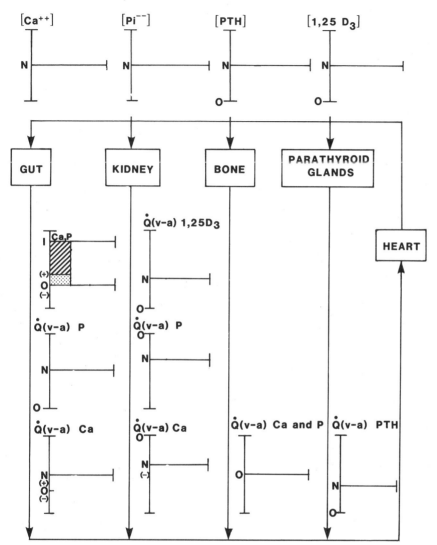

Figure 7–8. Normal regulation of minerals. Gut, kidney, bone, and parathyroid glands are shown as parallel processors of arterial blood. Arterial supply to the four organs is transformed for each of the materials as shown on the graphs. In the case of gut, delivery of calcium and phosphorus into the venous return, the product of flow (Q), and the venous (v) minus arterial (a) difference, is always above zero for phosphorus and may range from below to above zero for calcium. Fecal losses (striped bars) of calcium and phosphorus, when added to urinary losses (stippled bars), normally equal dietary intake (I) in stable and normal adults. In growing children their sum would be less than dietary intake. Delivery of phosphorus and calcium into renal venous blood is always set such that venous blood is relatively deficient in both minerals compared with arterial blood, so that there is net extraction and loss of the minerals into the urine. Delivery of $1,25D_3$ ranges from zero to positive values. Bone (Q) (v-a) for calcium and phosphorus may vary above and below zero but normally is at zero in the adult. Parathyroid hormone delivery into venous blood ranges from zero to a positive number. Normal blood values are schematized above the arterial inflow line for both hormones and both minerals of interest.

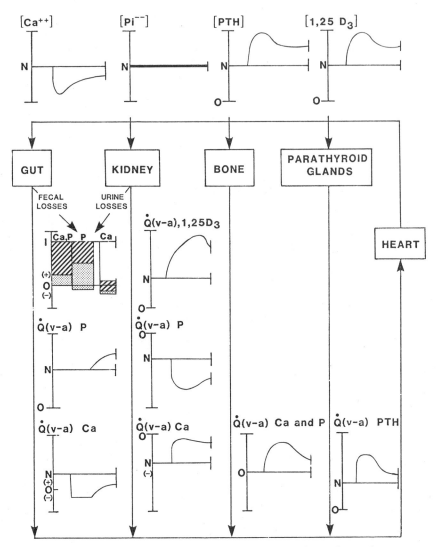

Figure 7–9. Response of mineral homeostatic regulation to low calcium diet. See text for details.

Calculations for the derivation of the "minimum daily requirement."

results except that bone mineral stores will be protected and mineral balances will be neutral, not negative. This value of D (Ca) is the minimum daily requirement (MDR), about 4 to 6 mg/kg/day for adults.

Growth. This state is one of chronically high β. Values of bone Q(v-a) are chronically below 0; [1,25(OH)$_2$D$_3$], [PTH], and portal Q(v-a) for Ca and P all are above adult normal, as in low calcium diet. The minimum daily requirement for calcium is higher because net absorption must always balance skeletal mineral demand.

Pregnancy and Lactation. For this state, Figure 7–8 must be modified to include the breasts or uterus with the other organs, with very negative values of Q(v-a) for Ca and P. This must be balanced by increased portal Q(v-a) for both, and this is accomplished by an elevated 1,25(OH)$_2$D$_3$ value. The mechanism of increased 1,25(OH)$_2$D$_3$ is in part increased [PTH] as in low calcium diet.

DISORDERS OF CALCIUM, PHOSPHORUS, AND MAGNESIUM

The clinical consequences of disordered mineral balance arise from abnormal serum mineral levels, which lead to bone disease and dysfunction of the nervous system, muscles, or kidneys, and from hypercalciuria that can produce renal stones. The disorders are classified as hypercalciuric and hypercalcemic states, hypocalcemic states, and states of excessive phosphate or magnesium loss (Tables 7–1 and 7–2) even though, as secondary consequences, all minerals may be abnormal in serum or urine in many of the conditions.

Hypercalcemic and Hypercalciuric States

Hyperabsorption. *Vitamin D Excess.* Excessive vitamin D_3 or $1,25(OH)_2D_3$ ingestion that raises serum $[1,25(OH)_2D_3]$ increases intestinal calcium and phosphorus absorption (Fig. 7–10); $1,25(OH)_2D_3$ excess is depicted, so serum $1,25(OH)_2D_3$ is shown as elevated. $1,25(OH)_2D_3$ production is reduced. Serum [Ca] and [P] are increased by hyperabsorption and PTH secretion and serum [PTH] are reduced. Low PTH decreases r(Ca) and bone mineral turnover, so $[Ca^{++}]$ comes under two opposing influences and is only mildly elevated. Low PTH increases r(P), however, so [P] is increased by both elevated absorption and tubule reabsorption. Fecal calcium and phosphorus losses are low,

Table 7–1. HYPERCALCEMIC AND HYPERCALCIURIC STATES

Name	Renal Stones	Serum				Urine
		Cr	Ca	P	PTH	Ca
		(mg/dl)				(mg/day)
Hyperabsorptive states						
Vitamin D excess[a]	(+)	↑	>12	↑	↓	400–800
Calcium excess	(+)		N	N		250–350
Increased bone resorption						
Malignant neoplasms[b]	(−)	↑	>14	↑	[c]	400–800
Immobilization	(+)	N	N	↑	↓	200–500
Paget's disease	(+)	N	N	N	N	300–400
Rapidly progressive osteo-porosis	(+)	N	N	N	N	300–400
Hyperthyroidism, glucocorticoid	(+)	N	<11	N	N	300–400
Abnormal renal reabsorption						
Increased[d]	(−)	±	<11	N	N	<200
Reduced[e]	(±)	±	N	N	−	300–400
Disorders with multiple defects						
Primary hyperparathyroidism	(+)	±	<14	↓	↑	300–500
Phosphate depletion	(−)	N	<11	↓	↓	300–400
Idiopathic hypercalciuria	(+)	N	N	±	↑ or ↓	300–500

[a]D_3 excess, $1,25(OH)_2D_3$ excess (sarcoid, pharmacologic)
[b]Epithelial tumor, myeloma, leukemia
[c]May be elevated by ectopic PTH production, otherwise low
[d]Familial hypocalciuric hypercalcemia (FHH), thiazide, ECTV depletion
[e]Lasix, distal RTA, Fanconi's syndrome, cystic medullary disease, Wilson's disease
Abbreviations: Cr, creatinine; Ca, calcium (mg/dl); P, phosphorus; PTH, serum PTH level; N, normal; ±, high or low; (+), Ccr; (−) do not occur.

Table 7–2. HYPOCALCIURIC, PHOSPHATURIC, AND MAGNESURIC STATES

Hypocalcemic states
    Reduced absorption
        Vitamin D deficiency: nutritional, vitamin D–dependent rickets
        Chronic renal failure
        Intestinal malabsorption
    Reduced PTH effects
        Hypoparathyroidism: surgical, primary, Mg deficiency
        Pseudohypoparathyroidism
        Rapid bone remineralization

Phosphaturic states
    VDRR
    Fanconi syndrome
    Post renal transplantation
    Mesenchymal tumors

Magnesuric states
    Alcoholism
    Ketoacidosis
    Drugs

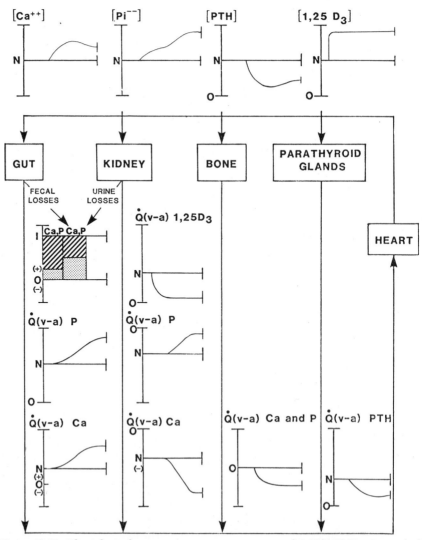

Figure 7–10. Physiological responses to primary excess of $1,25(OH)_2D_3$. See text for details.

but urine excretion rates of both are elevated and calcium renal stones may form.

The combination of increased [Ca] and [P] raises blood supersaturation with respect to calcium phosphate, and may promote crystal deposition in bone, kidney, blood vessels, heart, lungs, and elsewhere. Renal deposits are tubulointerstitial and can lower GFR. Elevated blood [Ca] itself also can lower GFR. As Eq. 5 shows, lower GFR must raise [Ca] and [P] unless r(Ca) and r(P) fall. r(P), especially, cannot fall very much, because PTH is low, and r(Ca) is already low, so a vicious cycle of renal damage, mounting hypercalcemia and hyperphosphatemia, and further renal damage can occur. In addition, increased [Ca^{++}] reduces distal nephron response to vasopressin, causing polyuria that can deplete ECF volume and thereby lower GFR and raise r(P) and r(Ca).

Vitamin D intoxication has serious, long-term consequences.

Clinically, vitamin D intoxication can cause severe renal damage. The worst problems occur with D$_3$ itself, because the material accumulates in the liver and may cause hyperabsorption for many weeks or months, whereas 1,25(OH)$_2$D$_3$ is metabolized very rapidly. Sarcoidosis may raise production of 1,25(OH)$_2$D$_3$, and does, rarely, cause hypercalcemic nephropathy. Hypercalciuria with very mild hypercalcemia is more common in sarcoid, and occurs mainly in patients with disseminated systemic involvement.

Treatment depends upon removing the source of excess hormone, maintaining a high level of urinary calcium and phosphorus excretion, and keeping calcium intake as low as possible. Intravenous saline infusion will raise GFR and favor excretion; furosemide can be used to reduce calcium reabsorption in the thick ascending limb of Henle's loop and foster its excretion. If serum levels are only moderately elevated (Ca<11; P<5) management may be on an outpatient basis.

Calcium Excess. Calcium antacids and extreme use of dairy products can raise Dα (Ca), but the increase (see Fig. 7–1) is small because any tendency to raise blood [Ca] lowers [PTH] and [1,25(OH)$_2$D$_3$], which in turn reduces α. At most, extreme calcium excess of many grams daily will raise urine calcium and may, possibly, cause kidney stones.

If high calcium intake is combined with even a modest excess of vitamin D$_3$, however, a picture of vitamin D intoxication may develop. If the calcium source is partly milk, which is rich in phosphorus as well as calcium, blood [Ca^{++}] × [P$^=$] may rise rapidly and create renal failure. Renal failure caused by excessive intake of milk, containing vitamin D$_3$ with calcium carbonate alkali, has been described as the *milk alkali syndrome.*

Increased Bone Resorption. Mineral absorption is normal or low in these conditions (Table 7–1), but bone Q(v-a) is elevated; the excess calcium lost from bone causes hypercalciuria and, when marked, hypercalcemia. The usual causes are epithelial tumors metastatic to bone from lung, breast, kidney, prostate, and thyroid, multiple myeloma, and some lymphomas. Less common causes, Paget's disease, immobilization, hyperthyroidism, glucocorticoid excess, and rapidly progressive osteoporosis, cause hypercalciuria but only mild and variable hypercalcemia.

Malignant Neoplasms. Malignant tumors cause severe hypercalciuria and probably are the most common reason for serious, life-threatening hypercalcemia. Rapid bone destruction is analogous to vitamin D intoxication in that $D(\alpha\text{-}\beta)$ rises; but the increase results from a large negative value for β, not an increase in α (Fig. 7–11). As in vitamin D excess, [PTH] is reduced; $[1,25(OH)_2D_3]$ will be lowered by low PTH and high $[Ca^{++}]$ and $[P^=]$. The low PTH lowers r(Ca), which is beneficial in promoting urine excretion of calcium and moderating hypercalcemia, but it also raises r(P), so hyperphosphatemia can be severe. As in vitamin D intoxication, an elevated $[Ca^{++}] \times [P^=]$ product promotes crystal deposition in kidney, lung, myocardium, cardiac conducting system, joints (producing apatite arthropathy), and blood vessels. Hypercalcemia itself, ECF volume depletion, decreased water reabsorption, and renal calcium phosphate tissue deposits all lower GFR, and falling GFR worsens both hypercalcemia and hyperphosphatemia.

The treatment of severe hypercalcemia from bone destruction is like that of vitamin D intoxication. Saline infusion and furosemide will

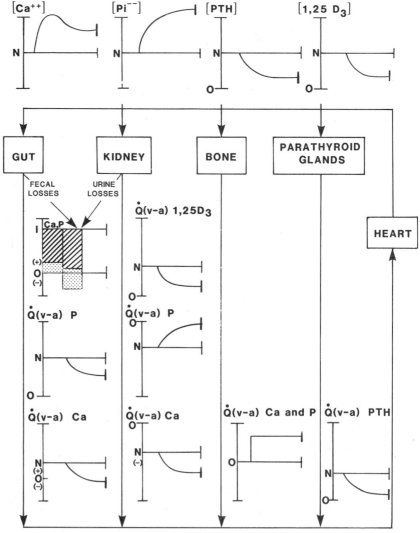

Figure 7–11. Pathophysiologic adjustments in states of increased bone reabsorption. See text for details.

promote calcium and phosphate losses in urine. Glucocorticoids can reduce bone mineral destruction, by multiple myeloma especially. Some tumors elaborate prostaglandins that promote bone dissolution, and indomethacin is helpful. The hormone calcitonin is useful in Paget's disease and malignant tumors, but is effective only transiently. Mithramycin may be effective but causes bone marrow suppression, thrombocytopenia, and occasionally liver and kidney damage.

Other Causes. Paget's disease, immobilization, rapidly progressive osteoporosis, hyperthyroidism, and glucocorticoid excess differ from malignant tumors in that bone $Q(v\text{-}a)$ rises less, the extra calcium and phosphorus are readily dissipated into the urine, and hypercalcemia and hyperphosphatemia are mild to absent. The usual manifestations are renal stones, because hypercalciuria may be chronic over many years; the bone disease itself produces diffuse osteopenia. Hyperthyroidism, glucocorticoid excess, and immobilization may be reversible conditions, but bone cannot be induced to remineralize completely after their treatment. Paget's disease can be treated using calcitonin, diphosphonate, and even mithramycin. Osteoporosis is not treatable at this time.

Abnormal Tubule Reabsorption. Increased Calcium Reabsorption. Thiazide diuretic agents raise distal tubule calcium reabsorption and, because $D(\alpha\text{-}\beta)$ does not decrease, serum calcium increases. The increase is small, for increased filtered load easily overbalances the increase in reabsorption. Rarely, tubule calcium reabsorption is increased by an inherited disorder called familial hypocalciuric hypercalcemia (FHH). The defect appears to be autosomal dominant; increased $r(Ca)$ may occur in the thick ascending limb. The biochemical pattern is identical to the thiazide effect, except that hypercalcemia may be more pronounced, in the range of 11 mg/dl. ECF volume depletion also raises $r(Ca)$ and may cause slight hypercalcemia.

Thiazide diuretic use gives the same clinical picture and has a nearly identical biochemical pattern to that of familial hypocalciuric hypercalcemia.

The clinical presentation of FHH is asymptomatic, mild hypercalcemia. Urine calcium and serum and urine phosphorus are normal. Serum PTH is normal, despite hypercalcemia. It is important to avoid parathyroid surgery, which is unnecessary and will not correct the hypercalcemia. Thiazide diuretic use gives the same clinical picture, but one must recheck serum calcium without the drug since another hypercalcemic state may be present. ECF volume depletion usually is obvious. Like thiazide, it may accentuate the hypercalcemia of another disorder, such as primary hyperparathyroidism, so follow-up measurements of serum calcium are necessary after volume depletion has been corrected.

Reduced Calcium Reabsorption. Calcium reabsorption is reduced by furosemide, probably because the drug inhibits its reabsorption by the thick ascending limb. Systemic response to furosemide has not been studied; whether PTH and $1,25(OH)_2D_3$ rise, and increased α offsets the excess urinary losses, is unknown. Chronic metabolic acidosis also reduces $r(Ca)$, perhaps in distal nephron segments, and causes hypercalciuria when GFR is normal. Since chronic metabolic acidosis and normal GFR coexist mainly when renal tubule proton excretion is defective (renal tubular acidosis, RTA), this is the main clinical example. In RTA of the hereditary distal type, hypercalciuria can cause stones, and osteomalacia may occur. Calcium balance may become negative at values of Dα sufficient to maintain positive balance in normal people, but this is not certain.

In proximal tubule disorders (Fanconi's syndrome), phosphate reabsorption is very reduced, producing phosphaturia and hypophosphatemia. Magnesuria is also present. Hypercalciuria is variable, perhaps because the thick ascending limb of Henle's loop and the distal tubule compensate for reduced proximal reabsorption. Cystic medullary disease and Wilson's disease also cause hypercalciuria, even when GFR is reduced. Taken together, Fanconi's syndrome, RTA, and the cystic diseases are extremely rare causes of osteomalacia or stones.

Disorders With Multiple Defects. *Primary Hyperparathyroidism.* In this clinical state PTH production is elevated chronically, but the pathogenesis is best presented as if PTH production were suddenly raised (Fig. 7–12). Serum [PTH] rises immediately; because the hormone acts rapidly upon kidney, r(P) and Q(v-a)P fall, and r(Ca),

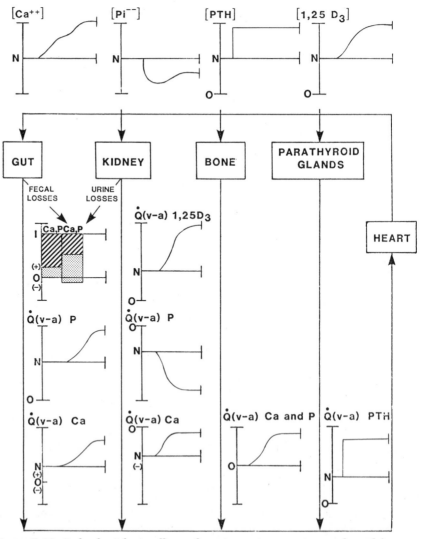

Figure 7–12. Pathophysiologic effects of a primary increase in parathyroid hormone (PTH).

$1,25(OH)_2D_3$ production, blood $[1,25(OH)_2D_3]$, and egress of calcium and phosphorus from bone all rise. The effects of PTH on bone and kidney raise blood [Ca], and lower [P]; low [P] further stimulates $1,25(OH)_2D_3$ production. Elevated $[1,25(OH)_2D_3]$ raises α, and blood [Ca] increases further, whereas serum phosphate comes under the opposing influences of hyperabsorption and the hypophosphatemic effects of reduced r(P). Urine calcium and phosphorus are increased both by increased absorption and bone resorption, and mineral balance is slightly negative.

The bone effects reflect PTH stimulation of surface osteoclasts, which proliferate and cause subperiosteal bone reabsorption. With time, osteocytes in the haversian canals also proliferate, enlarge the canals, and cause a diffuse cystic appearance of bone radiographically. The disease is called osteitis fibrosa cystica, because cell proliferation originally gave the mistaken appearance of inflammation, and fibrous connective tissue comes to replace cystic areas of bone.

Clinically, primary PTH overproduction is usually caused by adenoma or hyperplasia of the parathyroid glands; the former accounts for 85 percent of cases of primary hyperparathyroidism. Hypercalcemia, hypercalciuria, hypophosphatemia, and reduced r(P) are predictable (Fig. 7–12) and usual findings; serum PTH is elevated when a sensitive carboxy terminus assay is used; urine cAMP excretion is elevated. Many patients are symptomless and hypercalcemia is found by routine laboratory screening; others have renal stones, evidence of bone disease such as bone pain, fractures, elevated alkaline phosphatase, or abnormal radiographs, and, perhaps from hypercalcemia, peptic ulcer or pancreatitis, hypertension, and reduced GFR. In general, if the serum calcium is below 11 mg/dl and all manifestations of organ damage and stone are absent, one can postpone surgery unless a manifestation appears; otherwise, surgical cure by removal of the enlarged gland(s) is required.

Primary hyperparathyroidism is caused by adenoma in 85 percent of cases.

Diagnosis depends upon the presence of hypercalcemia, which is inevitably present, and exclusion of other hypercalcemic states. Vitamin D excess and sarcoid differ in their pathogenesis and manifestations (Fig. 7–10) and are clinically evident in most cases. Malignant tumors, especially hypernephroma and lung cancer, may produce material similar to PTH. Excess thyroid hormone may cause both hypercalcemia and hypercalciuria, but causes clinical stigmata of hyperthyroidism. Malignant neoplasms involving bone cause hypercalcemia, but are usually evident. Thiazide diuretics, ECF volume depletion, and familial hypocalciuric hypercalciuria are normocalciuric or hypocalciuric states of increased r(Ca) with mild hypercalcemia.

Phosphate Depletion. Though unusual in clinical practice, this is an important pathophysiologic model. Phosphate-binding antacids can produce it, as can nutritional deficiency such as occurs in alcoholism. Chronic hyperparathyroidism may also cause phosphate depletion. The first event is reduced intestinal Q(v-a)P and falling [P]; blood [Ca] rises because less calcium is in the form of calcium-phosphate complex, so PTH falls. Low [P] directly raises $1,25(OH)_2D_3$ production and blood $[1,25(OH)_2D_3]$. Low PTH and low [P] both can increase r(P), so renal Q(v-a)P rises and both factors also reduce r(Ca), so Q(v-a)Ca falls. Increased $[1,25(OH)_2D_3]$ raises intestinal Ca absorption and blood [Ca], and causes hypercalciuria. Bone is under two opposing influences in that low PTH reduces turnover, but low blood $[Ca^{++}] \times [P^=]$ favors dissolution. Chronically, the low $[Ca^{++}] \times [P^=]$ ion product produces osteomalacia, because newly formed osteoid cannot mineralize and trabecular surfaces become coated with unmineralized osteoid. In children, there are bone deformities and stunted growth, called rickets; in adults, bone pain occurs, with elevated alkaline phosphatase, fractures, and muscle weakness (osteomalacia).

Phosphate depletion may be a factor in primary hyperparathyroidism. Chronic low r(P) is offset by increased phosphate absorption, but low serum $[P^=]$ may reduce cell phosphate accumulation. Serum $1,25(OH)_2D_3$ may be raised by low P as well as PTH, worsening calcium hyperabsorption, and the expected increase of r(Ca) from PTH may be blunted by low [P], which reduces r(Ca). Low [P] also may reduce renal proton excretion and lead to hyperchloremic acidosis.

Idiopathic Hypercalciuria. This inherited condition of normocalciuria hypercalciuria seems to arise from an admixture of excessive $1,25(OH)_2D_3$ production and reduced r(Ca). It is a major cause of calcium renal stones.

Clinical Evaluation. Given routine serum measurements and urine calcium excretion, the various hypercalciuric and hypercalcemic states are not difficult to distinguish in their usual forms. Severe hypercalcemia (>12 mg/dl) is caused mainly by malignant tumors, vitamin D excess, and hyperparathyroidism; the latter is a hypophosphatemic state, azotemia is unusual, and calcium losses are not as severe as in the other two, which are easily differentiated clinically (Table 7–1). The normocalciuric or hypocalciuric states form a group of their own, and thiazide use or ECF volume depletion are clinically obvious.

Hypercalciuric and normocalcemic patients usually have idiopathic hypercalciuria. Paget's disease raises alkaline phosphatase and is radiologically detected. Immobilization, thyroid hormone, or glucocorticoid excess, and rapidly progressive osteoporosis are clinical diagnoses, as are use of furosemide or the presence of renal tubule defects or cystic renal diseases.

The wide distribution of abnormalities in hypercalciuria and hypercalcemia make diagnosis confusing and difficult.

However, confusion occurs because each of the disorders is not homogeneous but has a distribution of abnormalities. Sarcoid and vitamin D intoxication can cause normocalcemic hypercalciuria, which when mild is easily confused with idiopathic hypercalciuria. Though never absent, hypercalcemia in hyperparathyroidism may be very mild, and not properly appreciated. Mild hypercalcemia can occur in hyperabsorptive or bone-resorptive states, and be confused with hyperparathyroidism. The only guide in these overlapping conditions is careful clinical evaluation for each individual state; idiopathic hypercalciuria, the most common, is diagnosed by exclusion.

Hypocalcemic States

Reduced Absorption. *Vitamin D Deficiency.* Given adequate exposure to the sun, the skin can synthesize enough vitamin D_3 from cholesterol to preserve mineral nutrition; but in the northern countries vitamin D deficiency was common before the vitamin was added to milk, and still is not rare. Children are most susceptible because of their growth needs, as are elderly people, who have marginal diets and tend to remain indoors. Inadequate vitamin D nutrition can occur from intestinal fat malabsorption despite an adequate diet. Phenytoin can interfere with hepatic $25(OH)D_3$ production. There is a rare disorder, vitamin D-dependent rickets, type I, in which renal $1,25(OH)_2D_3$ production is inadequate despite normal serum $25(OH)_2D_3$ levels, and vitamin D_3 must be given to prevent functional consequences of $1,25(OH)_2D_3$ deficiency. In type II vitamin D-dependent rickets, $1,25(OH)_2D_3$ receptors appear defective, and $1,25(OH)_2D_3$ must be given in large amounts.

The pathophysiology of D deficiency can be described as though vitamin D supply suddenly was disrupted, although the disease is chronic. Absence of D_3 will lower blood $25(OH)D_3$, and both $1,25(OH)_2D_3$ production and blood level. Intestinal absorption of Ca, P, and Mg will fall. Calcium and magnesium absorption are more severely affected than that of phosphorus, perhaps because there are greater passive forces for phosphorus absorption. Hypocalcemia occurs and PTH production rises. High [PTH] reduces r(P), and along with reduced α(P) causes hypophosphatemia; PTH raises r(Ca). Urine Ca and P excretion rates both are low. Initially, high PTH raises bone Q(v-a) for Ca and P. Trabecular surfaces gradually become coated with unmineralized osteoid, however, because vitamin D is needed to promote mineralization and the low $[Ca^{++}] \times [P^=]$ product reduces the driving force for mineralization. Bone turnover and mineral loss therefore become low. Serum calcium is lowered by a low α(a) and Q(v-a)Ca. The clinical picture in children is rickets; in adults, osteomalacia.

Chronic Renal Failure. As nephrons are lost, $1,25(OH)_2D_3$ production is reduced by the loss of proximal convoluted tubule cells and intestinal absorption of Ca, P, and Mg falls (Fig. 7–13). Total GFR also falls, so serum $[Ca^{++}]$ and $[P^=]$ come under the two opposing influences of low absorption and low GFR. For calcium, the net result is a fall in serum level, which raises PTH secretion. Phosphorus absorption is better preserved, so that despite reduced α(P) and r(P) for PTH increase, blood $[P^=]$ tends to be increased. High [PTH] also raises Q(v-a)P from bone, which helps to maintain $[Ca^{++}]$ near normal, but tends to raise $[P^=]$ even more. $1,25(OH)_2D_3$ production is also under opposing influences: it is lowered by reduced nephron mass and slight increase of $[P^=]$, but raised by high [PTH] and low $[Ca^{++}]$; overall, it is below normal. This is a time of extraordinary dynamic equilibrium between the opposing forces of high PTH and low GFR and tubule mass, and is called a period of "compensated" renal failure.

Compensation eventually becomes impossible, because GFR falls so low that high PTH cannot reduce r(P) enough to prevent hyperphosphatemia. Progressive hyperphosphatemia reduces $1,25(OH)_2D_3$ production, and therefore calcium absorption, serum calcium, and α(P), but the fall in α(P) is never enough to keep blood $[P^=]$ from rising. As $1,25(OH)_2D_3$ falls, blood $[Ca^{++}]$ falls and [PTH] rises. The final result is chronic hypocalcemia, severe calcium malabsorption, high PTH, and low $1,25(OH)_2D_3$.

The effects of chronic renal failure on bone reflect PTH excess that causes osteitis fibrosa, and $1,25(OH)_2D_3$ deficiency that causes osteomalacia; the two lesions vary in relative severity depending upon the particular details of mineral balance in each patient. The initial

In chronic renal failure, excess PTH causes osteitis fibrosa, and $1,25(OH)_2D_3$ deficiency causes osteomalacia.

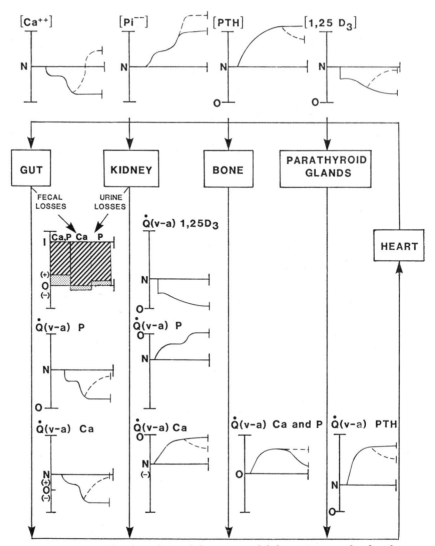

Figure 7–13. Pathophysiology of chronic renal failure. See text for details.

phase is principally a period of PTH excess combined with reduced but still significant $1,25(OH)_2D_3$ level, so osteitis fibrosa predominates. In the uncompensated phase, $1,25(OH)_2D_3$ deficiency becomes severe and osteomalacia may predominate if unmineralized osteoid eventually covers all trabecular surfaces and prevents osteocytes from removing bone mineral.

The administration of $1,25(OH)_2D_3$ creates an instructive pathophysiologic model that is of clinical interest now that the hormone is available for oral administration. Intestinal calcium and phosphorus absorption rise to normal, but GFR remains low. $[P^=]$ and $[Ca^{++}]$ must therefore rise, unless measures such as low phosphorus diet and oral phosphate-binding agents are used to prevent phosphorus absorption. $1,25(OH)_2D_3$ also permits osteoid to mineralize, and high PTH then permits osteitis fibrosa to progress, so bone Q[v-a] must rise (dashed lines, Fig. 7–13). As $[Ca^{++}]$ rises, [PTH] may fall, but only slightly, because very chronic PTH overproduction causes all four glands to become very large, 10- to 100-fold above normal, and parathyroid cells cannot reduce PTH production to zero. So even as $[Ca^{++}]$ becomes supranormal, and each cell secretes at its basal rate, the product of cell number $\times$ rate/cell remains high (Fig. 7–12, dashed lines). As a result, r(Ca) is stimulated by PTH, D (α-β) for calcium is elevated by $1,25(OH)_2D_3$, and $[Ca^{++}] \times [P^=]$ can rise above normal.

The final result, hyperphosphatemia and elevated $[Ca^{++}]$, is reminiscent of vitamin D intoxication because $[Ca^{++}] \times [P^=]$ can be elevated enough that soft tissue calcification occurs. In a sense, $1,25(OH)_2D_3$ at even normal levels can be excessive in chronic renal failure because PTH secretion is elevated and phosphate retention difficult to avoid. Even if PTH secretion were normal, phosphate retention would still pose hazards unless its absorption were reduced. The combination of measures to reduce P absorption, parathyroidectomy and $1,25(OH)_2D_3$ repletion, is a basis for treatment.

Intestinal Malabsorption. There are two ways for malabsorption to influence mineral balance. Fat malabsorption from pancreatic insufficiency or biliary obstruction can lower vitamin D absorption and, in northern latitudes particularly, can cause nutritional D deficiency. Alternatively, intestinal epithelial cell absorption can be insufficient despite adequate vitamin D, because of extensive small bowel resection or damage by diseases such as regional enteritis or small bowel infarction. In either case, Q(v-a)Ca and P fall but, as usual, calcium absorption is the more severely affected. The pathophysiology is that of extreme low calcium diet (Fig. 7–9) combined with phosphate depletion. The clinical picture in children is rickets and in the adult is osteomalacia and muscle weakness. Magnesium malabsorption also occurs, causing hypomagnesemia that may blunt PTH response and worsen hypocalcemia. Combined hypocalcemia and hypomagnesemia can cause tetany.

Reduced PTH Effects. *Hypoparathyroidism.* The lack of PTH causes a picture that is the exact inverse of hyperparathyroidism. Renal $1,25(OH)_2D_3$ and r(Ca) are low, r(P) is high, and intestinal absorption of calcium and phosphate are low, as is bone turnover. The results are hypocalcemia and hyperphosphatemia. Attempts to increase blood $[Ca^{++}]$ by oral calcium load or $1,25(OH)_2D_3$ administration causes marked hypercalciuria because r(Ca) is low and $[Ca^{++}]$ can become normal only at very high levels of D(α)Ca. Phosphate absorption is also stimulated by $1,25(OH)_2D_3$ and r(P) is elevated by low PTH, so the $[Ca^{++}] \times [P^=]$ product can become elevated. In other words, it is easy to produce vitamin D intoxication. This illustrates how crucial PTH is in down-regulating serum $[P^=]$ when phosphate absorption rises. Here, there is no PTH and r(P) is fixed at a maximal level.

The main problems in hypoparathyroidism are paresthesia or tetany from hypocalcemia, and the main goal of treatment is to keep [Ca] high enough to prevent symptoms without provoking tissue damage from high $[Ca^{++}] \times [P^=]$ or producing such severe hypercalciuria that renal stones occur. The best approach is to raise r(Ca) using a thiazide diuretic agent, which stimulates distal tubule calcium reabsorption. Then, modest calcium supplementation of 1 to 2 gm of calcium daily (as calcium lactate, calcium carbonate, or calcium gluconate) in 3 to 4 divided doses, very small amounts of $1,25(OH)_2D_3$, or a sterol analogue such as dihydroxytachysterol, which raises α(Ca), should

Osteomalacia and muscle weakness can result from extensive small bowel resection, because calcium absorption is severely reduced.

suffice to raise $[Ca^{++}]$ without unduly raising phosphate absorption. The ideal drug that also lowers r(P) is not yet known.

Pseudohypoparathyroidism. This rare disorder exists in multiple forms; the main problem in each is that kidney or bone cells fail to respond to PTH. In general, the pathophysiology is like that of PTH deficiency, but a detailed analysis of any one patient requires a dissection of bone and renal responsiveness. Subtypes and approaches to treatment are discussed in more specialized texts.

"Hungry bone syndrome" can require urgent treatment.

Rapid Bone Remineralization. Within hours after successful cure of longstanding hyperparathyroidism (by parathyroidectomy), bone may rapidly reaccumulate calcium, phosphorus, and magnesium *(hungry bone syndrome)*. This also can occur with sudden treatment of chronic hypophosphatemic osteomalacia. Blood $[Ca^{++}]$, $[P^=]$, and $[Mg^+]$ all fall and cause hypocalcemic hypomagnesemic tetany; low Mg prevents remaining parathyroid glands from secreting PTH in response to low $[Ca^{++}]$, so there is no mechanism for systemic compensation.

This condition can be a medical emergency because of tetany and laryngospasm. Treatment is with intravenous calcium chloride or gluconate and magnesium. An infusion of calcium is given for the ensuing several days, along with oral calcium and $1,25(OH)_2D_3$. As [Ca] rises, oral dosages are adjusted and parenteral treatment discontinued.

Phosphaturic States. *Hereditary Vitamin D-Resistant Rickets (VDRR).* In this condition renal tubule phosphate reabsorption, r(P), is reduced and there is severe hypophosphatemia, low $[Ca^{++}] \times [P^=]$, and rickets or osteomalacia. Serum [Ca], urine calcium excretion, serum PTH and, surprisingly, $1,25(OH)_2D_3$ levels are normal. Given the extremely high $1,25(OH)_2D_3$ level of phosphate depletion, despite low [PTH], one must conclude that the syndrome produces hypophosphatemia but not the usual renal cell response to phosphate depletion. The clinical picture is described by the name. Treatment with 1 to 2 gm daily of elemental phosphate, orally, can heal the bone lesion.

Post-transplantation Hypophosphatemia. Low r(P) with hypophosphatemia is common in transplanted kidneys; serum $[Ca^{++}]$ and urine calcium are both normal, as in VDRR, and osteomalacia may occur. The lack of hypercalciuria suggests that $1,25(OH)_2D_3$ is not elevated, but the matter has not been studied in detail. Treatment as in VDRR is effective in preventing bone disease.

This disorder must be distinguished from persistent hyperparathyroidism, which also lowers blood $[P^=]$ and r(P). Excess PTH tends to produce hypercalcemia, elevated serum $1,25(OH)_2D_3$ level, hypercalciuria, and high [PTH], whereas phosphate-wasting causes mainly hypophosphatemia.

Fanconi's Syndrome. Part of the hereditary or acquired syndrome of proximal tubule dysfunction is low r(P) and hypophosphatemia. It is differentiated from VDRR by the coexistence of aminoaciduria, glucosuria, hyperuricosuria with hypouricemia, and proximal renal tubule acidosis, and from hyperparathyroidism by normocalcemia. In this syndrome, there may be hypercalciuria caused by a tubule defect of calcium reabsorption or elevated $1,25(OH)_2D_3$; the latter is, as yet, unstudied.

Tumor-Induced Phosphaturia. Benign nonossifying mesenchymal tumors, often arising in soft tissues near bone, cause a condition of severely reduced r(P), hypophosphatemia, and osteomalacia, despite normocalcemia and normocalciuria. There is no other evidence of proximal tubule dysfunction. Treatment requires removal of the tumors, which is followed by rapid bone remineralization and healing of osteomalacia.

Magnesuric States. Hyperparathyroidism and vitamin D excess both can cause magnesuria, but it is incidental and does not cause clinical manifestations. However, alcoholism, diabetic ketoacidosis, malnutrition, malabsorption, and primary aldosteronism can cause significant urinary magnesium losses. Because intestinal absorption may be normal or even low, cell depletion of magnesium and hypomagnesemia may occur. The result may be muscle weakness and rhabdomyolysis, low PTH secretion with hypocalcemia, hypomagnesemia, and even tetany. Treatment is by parenteral magnesium repletion.

Significant urinary magnesium losses may accompany alcoholism, malnutrition, diabetic ketoacidosis, malabsorption, and primary aldosteronism.

REFERENCES

Normal Metabolism

Human and Animal Studies of Mineral Absorption

Lemann, J., Jr., Adams, N. D., and Gray, R. W.: Urinary calcium excretion in human beings. N. Engl. J. Med. 301:535–541, 1979.
A review of the factors that influence urinary calcium excretion. Increase in dietary calcium, acid, sodium but not phosphate increases urine calcium excretion.

Levine, B. S., Walling, M. W., and Coburn, J. W.: Effect of vitamin D sterols and dietary magnesium on calcium and phosphorus homeostasis. Am. J. Physiol. 241:E35–E41, 1981.
In vitamin D-deficient rats increasing dietary magnesium lowered intestinal calcium and phosphorus absorption. Treatment with 1,25(OH)₂D₃ overcame the decrease in absorption. Argument is made for two different mechanisms for calcium and phosphorus absorption, one vitamin D-dependent and the other vitamin D-independent.

Levine, B. S., Brautbar, N., Walling, M. W., Lee, D. B. N., and Coburn, J. W.: Effects of vitamin D and diet magnesium on magnesium metabolism. Am. J. Physiol. 239:E515–E523, 1980.
1,25 vitamin D₃ increased magnesium absorption and urine magnesium in vitamin D-deficient rats but did not alter magnesium balance or serum magnesium.

Segmental Intestinal Absorption

Norman, D. A., Fordtran, J. S., Brinkley, L. J., Zerwekh, J. E., Nicar, M. J., Strowig, S. M., and Pak, C. Y. C.: Jejunal and ileal adaptation to alterations in dietary calcium: Changes in calcium and magnesium absorption and pathogenetic role of parathyroid hormone and 1,25-dihydroxyvitamin D. J. Clin. Invest. 67:1599–1603, 1981.
Segments of jejunum and ileum were perfused in humans to assess calcium absorption in response to changes in dietary calcium. Low calcium diet stimulated calcium absorption in both segments; however, ileum responded more rapidly and more completely than jejunum.

Favus, M. J., Kathpalia, S. C., Coe, F. L., and Mond, A. E.: Effects of diet calcium and 1,25-dihydroxyvitamin D₃ on colon calcium active transport. Am. J. Physiol. 238:G75–G78, 1980.
Descending colon calcium transport response to diet calcium and 1,25(OH)₂D₃ were studied using Ussing chambers. Both low calcium diet and 1,25(OH)₂D₃ increased net calcium absorption by increasing the mucosal to serosal flux without altering the serosal to mucosal flux.

Cellular Mechanisms of Absorption

Murer, H., and Hildmann, B.: Transcellular transport of calcium and inorganic phosphate in the small intestinal epithelium. Am. J. Physiol. 240:G409–G416, 1981.
A review of intestinal calcium and phosphate transport. Models for active basolateral calcium and brush border phosphate transport are demonstrated. The roles for sodium exchange and 1,25(OH)₂D₃ activity are illustrated (55 references).

Berner, W., Kinne, R., and Murer, H.: Phosphate transport into brush-border membrane vesicles isolated from rat small intestine. Biochem. J. 160:467–474, 1976.
Phosphate transport was studied using brush border membrane vesicles from rat small intestine.

Regulation of $1,25(OH)_2D_3$ Production

Eisman, J. A., Prince, R. L., Wark, J. D., and Moseley, J. M.: Modulation of plasma 1,25-dihydroxyvitamin D in man by stimulation and suppression tests. Lancet 2:931–933, 1979.
In normal patients parathyroid hormone infusion led to a marked increase while an oral calcium load decreased the level of plasma $1,25(OH)_2D_3$.

Rasmussen, H., Wong, M., Bikle, D., and Goodman, D. B. P.: Hormonal control of the renal conversion of 25-hydroxycholecalciferol to 1,25-dihydroxycholecalciferol. J. Clin. Invest. 51:2502–2504, 1972.
Isolated renal tubules from vitamin D-deficient chicks were used to study the conversion of 25 hydroxyvitamin D_3 to 1,25 dihydroxyvitamin D_3. Bovine parathyroid hormone and cyclic AMP stimulated while calcitonin suppressed the conversion.

Tubule Reabsorption of Calcium, Phosphorus, and Magnesium

Sutton, R. A. L., and Dirks, J. H.: Calcium and magnesium: Renal handling and disorders of metabolism. *In* Brenner, B. M., and Rector, F. C., Jr., eds.: The Kidney. 3rd Edition. W. B. Saunders Co., Philadelphia, 1986.

Jacobson, H., and Knochel, J. P.: Renal handling of phosphate in health and disease. *In* Brenner, B. M., and Rector, F. C., Jr., eds.: The Kidney. 3rd Edition. W. B. Saunders Co., Philadelphia, 1986.
Comprehensive and current reviews.

Disorders of Calcium, Phosphorus, and Magnesium

Hypercalcemic and Hypercalciuric States

Paterson, C. R.: Vitamin-D poisoning: Survey of causes in 21 patients with hypercalcaemia. Lancet 1:1164–1165, 1980.
Vitamin D intoxication resulted in severe hypercalcemia in 21 patients; 2 patients died as a result. Caution is advised in treating patients with this hormone.

Orwoll, E. S.: The milk alkali syndrome—current concepts. Ann. Intern. Med. 97:242–248, 1982.
A recent review of the clinical aspects of the milk alkali syndrome. The differentiation from hyperparathyroidism is stressed. In general, discontinuation of the calcium and alkali results in rapid recovery.

Stewart, A. F., Horst, R., Deftos, L. J., et al.: Biochemical evaluation of patients with cancer-associated hypercalcemia: Evidence for humoral and nonhumoral groups. N. Engl. J. Med. 303:1377–1383, 1980.
Of 50 consecutive patients with cancer-associated hypercalcemias, 41 were found to have elevated urinary cyclic AMP excretion. When compared with 15 patients with primary hyperparathyroidism, the elevated cyclic AMP group had a similar reduction in tubule phosphorus threshold, but greater urinary calcium excretion, and a reduction of $1,25(OH)_2D_3$ and immunoreactive PTH. These data suggest that some patients with cancer-associated hypercalcemia have a serum factor that shares some properties of PTH, but is not native 1–84 PTH.

Heath, H., III, Earll, J. M., Schaaf, J. T., et al.: Serum ionized calcium during bed rest in fracture patients and normal men. Metabolism 21:633–640, 1972.
An elevation of ionized calcium was found in 9 of 10 patients immobilized for fracture treatment while an elevation of total calcium was found in only 3 of 10. Four normal control patients were placed at bed rest for 12 days. Total calcium remained normal; however, ionized calcium became elevated. The cause of the elevated calcium was not clear.

Kaye, M.: The effects in the rat of varying intakes of dietary calcium, phosphorus, and hydrogen ion on hyperparathyroidism due to chronic renal failure. J. Clin. Invest. 53:256–269, 1974.
Renal insufficiency of four weeks duration in rats led to parathyroid gland enlargement and increased bone resorption. Increasing phosphate intake and alkalosis led to parathyroid gland enlargement while increasing calcium intake and acidosis led to small parathyroid glands. In all cases, parathyroid gland weight was inversely related to ionized calcium.

Abnormal Tubule Reabsorption

Stole, R. M., Smith, C. H., Wilson, D. M., et al.: Hydrochlorothiazide effects on serum calcium and immunoreactive parathyroid hormone concentrations: Studies in normal subjects. Ann. Intern. Med. 77:587–591, 1972.
Nine normal subjects were given hydrochlorothiazide. Total and ionized calcium increased; however, there was no change in the level of immunoreactive parathyroid hormone.

Marx, S. J., Spiegel, A. M., Brown, E. M., et al.: Family studies in patients with primary parathyroid hyperplasia. Am. J. Med. 62:698–706, 1977.
The clinical and biochemical features of familial hypocalciuric hypercalcemia are discussed. In general, the prognosis is good and the disease requires no treatment. It must be differentiated from hyperparathyroidism because subtotal parathyroidectomy will not result in normalization of serum calcium in this disorder.

Suki, W. N., Yium, J. J., Von Hinden, et al.: Acute treatment of hypercalemia with furosemide. N. Engl. J. Med., 283:836–840, 1970.
The use of intravenous furosemide in the acute treatment of hypercalcemia is reviewed. In eight patients the mean fall in serum calcium was 3.1 mg caused by urine calcium loss of between 0.7 and 2.7 gm. Sodium, potassium, and magnesium losses are considerable and must be replaced.

Reiss, E., and Canterbury, J. M.: Spectrum of hyperparathyroidism. Am. J. Med. 56:794–799, 1974.
Hyperparathyroidism is defined as any condition associated with a persistently elevated level of circulating parathyroid hormone. Three groups are discussed: hypercalcemic, normocalcemic, and hypocalemic. Renal disease can be found in each of the groups.

Marx, S. J., Spiegel, A. M., and Levine, M. A., et al.: Familial hypocalciuric hypercalcemia: The relation to primary parathyroid hyperplasia. N. Engl. J. Med. 307:416–426, 1982.
The difference among familial hypocalciuric hypercalcemia, multiple endocrine neoplasias type I and II, and sporadic hyperparathyroidism are described. Familial hypocalciuric hypercalcemia exhibits autosomal dominant inheritance, nephrolithiasis and peptic ulcer disease are unusual, and subtotal parathyroidectomy was without benefit. With multiple endocrine neoplasia type I, high concentrations of glucagon were usually found and elevations of gastrin in 3 of 12.

Hypocalcemic States

Habener, J. F., and Mahaffely, J. E.: Osteomalacia and disorders of vitamin D metabolism. Ann. Rev. Med. 29:327–342, 1978.
The pathogenesis and clinical spectrum of osteomalacia is reviewed and its relationship to our understanding of vitamin D is discussed. Defects in the hydroxylation and target tissue action of vitamin D are reviewed.

Brickman, A. S., Coburn, J. W., and Massry, S. G.: 1,25-dihydroxy-vitamin D_3 in normal man and patients with renal failure. Ann. Intern. Med. 80:161–168, 1974.
The effects of oral treatment with $1,25(OH)_2D_3$ on calcium phosphorus metabolism in humans is reviewed. $1,25(OH)_2D_3$ increased calcium absorption in normal as well as uremic subjects. Uremic patients had an increase in serum calcium; effects on serum phosphate were variable.

Reduced PTH Effects

Breslau, N. A., and Pak, C. Y. C.: Hypoparathyroidism. Metabolism 28:1261–1276, 1979.
Hypoparathyroidism, its pathogenesis, classification, and management are discussed. Hypoparathyroidism may result from deficiency, ineffectiveness, or resistance to PTH. $1,25(OH)_2D_3$ is produced in subnormal amounts either because of a decrease in active PTH or the lack of hypophosphatemia. Treatment with vitamin D analogue is discussed.

Chase, L. R., Melson, G. L., and Aurbach, G. D.: Pseudohypoparathyroidism: Defective excretion of 3′,5′-AMP in response to parathyroid hormone. J. Clin. Invest. 48:1832–1844, 1969.
In patients with pseudohypoparathyroidism there is an abnormally high concentration of circulating parathyroid hormone that could be suppressed by hypercalcemia. Infusion of purified PTH did not result in an increase in excretion of cyclic adenosine 3′,5′-monophosphate as it did in controls.

Drezner, M., Neelson, F. A., and Lebovitz, H. E.: Pseudohypoparathyroidism type II: A possible defect in the reception of the cyclic AMP signal. N. Engl. J. Med. 289:1056–1060, 1973.
A case is described in which there is an excess of circulating PTH: Infusion of parathyroid hormone increases urinary cyclic AMP; however, there was no renal tubule response in terms of phosphate handling nor was there a rise in serum calcium. A defect appears to be in the intracellular reception of the second messenger, cyclic adenosine monophosphate.

Phosphaturic States

Glorieux, F. H., Marie, P. J., Pettifor, J. M., et al.: Bone response to phosphate salts, ergocalciferol, and calcitrol in hypophosphatemic vitamin D-resistant rickets. N. Engl. J. Med. 303:1023–1031, 1980.
Children with vitamin D-resistant rickets were treated with phosphate alone or combined with vitamin D_2 or $1,25(OH)_2D_3$. The combined regimen of $1,25(OH)_2D_3$ and phosphate did not correct the renal phosphate leak but led to an improved mineralization of trabecular bone. The most common complication, that of hypercalcemia, was easily controlled by adjustment of the $1,25(OH)_2D_3$ dose.

Magnesuric States

Mendelson, J. H., Borner, B., Mayman, C., et al.: The determination of exchangeable magnesium in alcoholic patients. Metabolism 14:88–98, 1965.
Exchangeable magnesium and urine loss of injected magnesium were both decreased in tremulous alcoholic patients. The defect of magnesium was thought to be secondary to poor dietary intake and intercurrent illnesses. A causal relationship between bone magnesium levels and tremulousness was not found.

Index

Page numbers in *italic* type indicate illustrations; page numbers followed by t refer to tables.

185